Timeless Beauty

Timeless Beauty

THE SECRET SCIENCE OF
BEAUTIFUL SKIN BEYOND 40

Marina Vashkevich

ISBN-13: 9781535411844
ISBN-10: 1535411848
Library of Congress Control Number: 2016911822
CreateSpace Independent Publishing Platform
North Charleston, South Carolina
Illustrations by Alex Vashkevich
Front-cover photography by Sasha Green
Cover design by Luba Chernyavsky

Contents

Foreword

Women in their forties and fifties typically face significant changes in their lives. They characteristically shift away from taking care of others to being free to take care of themselves. But they can also find themselves facing the *added* challenges of the effects of aging.

As a homeopathic doctor, I see the impact that these challenges have on women. Sleep, weight, hormone, and skin issues are common during this transition. They can cause great stress. This is what I treat.

Marina also understands these challenges and treats a wide range of skin issues that can arise during this time. She has extensive experience and an excellent ability to find a solution to these issues. This book reflects her deep understanding of this stage of women's lives.

Carol Jones, DHom, HMC
Toronto, Ontario, Canada
homeopathcarol@rogers.com

Preface

Hello, my name is Marina Vashkevich. I am a dermatologist in Belarus and the founder of MedVspa clinics in Europe, the United States, and Canada. I created these clinics because I was seeing the same approach and the same technology being used everywhere to treat skin ailments. Over my years of experience, I discovered that there was more to rejuvenating the skin than using one technology. So I created a unique combination of treatment protocols never seen in the industry before with maximum results to make my patients years younger. I am a dermatologist in Belarus and an international speaker at aesthetic-medicine conferences, and this has helped me develop my own view on the aging process.

My decision to be an aesthetic dermatologist was a pretty unexpected one for my colleagues and family. After graduating medical school in Belarus, I worked as a psychiatrist, and for fifteen years, I rescued drug-addicted teenagers.

Every medical doctor who has had the experience of working with drug-addicted teenagers will confirm that emotionally you won't be able to stay in this field for long. It was unbearable watching, every day, as how amazing, beautiful people passed away because of an overdose; how twins, the only sons of their mother, were sent to prison for many years because they were drug dealers; and how parents wishing their drug-addicted kids would die because they were not able to bear seeing how horrible their children were becoming. After fifteen years, I could not handle it anymore, and I decided I wanted to start helping people in other ways.

My unhappy circumstances created a physical problem. I became sick and went through a series of back surgeries. Recovery was horrible with lots of pain and 100 percent dependency on the people around me. It was impossible to sit on a chair or even lift my leg up onto a step. The three months that I spent in different hospitals gave me the time to think about what I should do in this life. This became a priceless treasure for me. I finally answered this question; I wanted to be an aesthetic dermatologist for my twentieth year as a doctor. It was now or never! Realizing this helped me to recover.

My dermatology residency was a thousand kilometers from my home city. I was not able to sit properly, carry something that weighed more than six pounds, or walk a thousand steps, and my brain was impaired by painkillers, but I was the happiest I had been. It seems that struggle followed me twelve hours per day. I took the extended program. I learned, watched, and asked questions. I remember being hungry for knowledge about the skin, dermatology, creams, technologies, fillers, and so on. This continued for three years. I never had a free weekend or time to read for fun or watch movies. The most interesting things to read for me were scientific dermatology books and magazines. I remember my first job; I asked everyone everything, and like a sponge, I absorbed everyone's knowledge and experience. People shared generously, and I looked at them with such hungry but sparkling eyes, asking for knowledge.

One year later, while participating in a dermatology class discussion, I started to answer the doctors' questions instead of them answering mine. Immediately, I was recruited by Viora, a world leader and manufacturer of skin-care technology systems in the United States and Europe, and was offered a contract for the clinical trials of their new system, which at the time was called Reaction. I was happy and excited. It predetermined my next step. I opened my own practice and started to take clients, work with them directly, evaluate results, optimize protocols, and build new protocols for the treatments, combining technologies, injections, and chemical peels. I have seen wrinkles disappear, faces lifted, and skin restored to its youthful glow. It was real happiness to make people's dreams a reality!

My experience was mentioned by many of my colleagues around the world, and I was invited to conferences as a speaker in Asia, the Middle East, Europe, and Russia. I talked about my hands-on experience in treating acne, getting rid of wrinkles and double chins, performing eye lifts, and shrinking excess skin after extreme weight loss. I combined technologies and built my own protocols.

But it was not enough. North America lured me in with its outstanding medical experience. I left my Belarus clinic in the hands of one of my top practitioners and moved my family to Canada.

I started my business eight months after coming to Canada, and a year later, I opened a location in the United States.

My clients inspired me not only to open a clinic in Bloor-Yorkville, Toronto, but also to write a book. All that you find in this book is my hands-on international experience. It is my consultation approach—everything that I discuss with the client during consultation. These are my conclusions, based on the most up-to-date knowledge in the field of international aesthetic medicine.

It is never too late to start something from the beginning, whatever your age. It is never too late to seize your passion and, for once in your life, do something that you have always dreamed about doing.

I am happy to present this book to you. I want to share my happiness with the results that I see. I want you to stop spending hours searching the Internet and reading about aging, your neck, and cellulite. I explain everything to you the way I do to my clients. What you will discover in this book will save you time and money and give you a new perspective on life. You can look years younger; there are combinations of technologies and treatments that can help, and I will show you how.

I am a very happy person now, and I am happy that I found the time, stopped, looked around, and shared everything that I know with you to make you happier. Welcome to the magic of aesthetic medicine!

Disclaimer

Please note that much of the information in this book is based on my personal experience and educational background as a medical doctor in dermatology in Belarus. Your particular situation may not be exactly suited to the examples illustrated in the book. You can use this information as you see fit, adjusting recommendations according to your particular situation and at your own risk.

Any trademarks, service marks, product names, or named features are assumed to be property of their respective owners and are used only for reference. There is no implied endorsement.

Please note that the information presented on these pages is for informational purposes only. The author shall not be liable to anyone for any loss or injury caused in whole or in part by your use of this information or for any decision you make or action you take relying on information you received from this text. This text is not intended to replace legal, medical, aesthetic, or other professional advice and is only meant to be used as a guideline for the reader.

Introduction

This book is dedicated to all of you who would like to live a long, vibrant life, enjoying your own natural beauty, using integrated and unique noninvasive solutions to help you age gracefully. What you will find in these pages will give you the secrets to looking five to ten years younger with a natural, never artificial, appearance. It's an enhancement and rejuvenation of your very own beauty.

Learn to smile at yourself in the mirror again like you used to ten years ago. There are many ways to make this happen, starting with modern technologies and injections.

This book gives you a clear explanation of why and how the aging process works and how to fight it while still maintaining a natural look.

I will let you know the secrets I've discovered, which are the most updated combinations of technologies, techniques, and injections that are able to give fantastic and long-lasting results.

In this book, you will find information that will save you lots of money and will give you the knowledge to know what to ask for and what to expect if you are going into a medical spa or clinic.

After reading this book, you will know exactly what type of aging you have, what the signs of your aging are, and what kind of technologies and injections will be able to give you the results that you really want.

The book is written for people looking for knowledge in the beauty industry, both customers and professionals.

CHAPTER 1

Simple Beauty instead of Long Internet Searches...

Have you ever wondered why the same techniques or technologies (systems, injections, or surgeries) that were applied to correct your aging process give fast and visible results without side effect for some people but are ineffective with a long downtime for others?

Bad results that do not satisfy a client are the result of a mistake in the diagnosis of the aging process. Aging is a multilevel process (skin, fat, veins, arteries, lymphatic vessels, bones, and muscles).

In Europe, we've named this field aesthetic medicine. *Aesthetics* means beauty. The practice of medicine includes a comprehensive approach, starting with assessment and diagnosis.

The right diagnosis and comprehensively evaluated plan of treatment will be able to correct the signs of aging in a natural way, using the natural potential of the body. It is the same as using a reserve of muscles to create body shape or using the right prescriptions to treat a disease.

In this book, I want you to understand what the right beauty diagnosis is for you. I will explain to you the simple way aesthetic medicine approaches and handles the symptoms of aging and help you to understand the newest methods available to help you keep your beauty for a long time with predictable results. I want you to age gracefully, and I will show you how.

Everything that you find in this book is based on my hands-on professional experience as a European (Belarus) dermatologist. This book offers many opinions from gurus in the field of aesthetic medicine. But all conclusions, opinions, and suggestions are my own secrets that I want to share with you.

If you would like to clarify something especially important for you, please contact me at marina@medvspa.com.

CHAPTER 2

The Successful Battle with Aging–Aging Types

Aesthetic medicine is different from the beauty industry. One of the most important aspects of modern aesthetic medicine is the necessity of building upon the diagnosis. The right diagnosis helps practitioners and clients to choose the best approach to treatment. Let's start with the diagnosis of the type of aging.

What Is Your Aging Type?

The aging process appears differently and varies from one person to another.[1]

1 I. I. Kolgunenko, *Gerontius Cosmetology* (1974).

There are four basic types of aging and one that combines all.

- **Sagging**
- **Tired**
- **Deformed**
- **Muscular**
- **Combination of types**

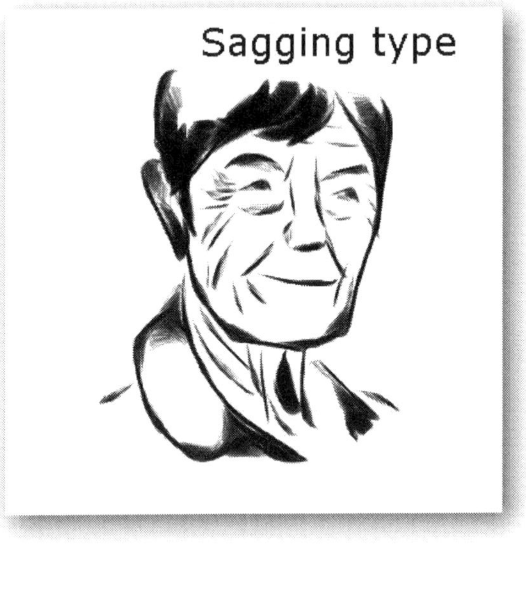

Types of Aging: Sagging

Lean, skinny people experience this type of aging. When they are younger, their skin looks perfect, even and smooth. In their twenties, representatives of this type complain that their skin is dry. In their thirties, they begin to notice the first wrinkles, usually around the eyes.

With age, skin gets covered by many shallow wrinkles caused by changes in the collagen structure. Collagen is the structural support of the skin. It consists of spirals. External factors like sun, sugar consumption, and age make it limp with the appearance of collagen-spiral cross-links. When cross-linked collagen is not able to play its supportive role in the skin structure, we see the changes as wrinkles and skin sagginess.

Around the age of fifty, the first deep lines show up, like deep wrinkles around the mouth. Signs of sun damage, like broken capillaries and dark spots, are more visible on faces with the sagging type of aging when compared with other types. All these changes take place because of decreasing skin elasticity and dehydration.

Many Caucasians are predisposed to this type of aging. It is explained by low levels of a skin-hydration factor, called natural moisturizing factor (NMF). It is not developed as well as in people of other ethnic groups. Lack of deep tissue hydration is a significant factor predisposing people to the emergence of wrinkles.

One more factor is sun. The sun's ultraviolet rays force the process of aging. That is why representatives of light skin types show the signs of aging faster, compared with other ethnic groups.

Treatment Plan for the Sagging Type

The treatment protocol should be focused on skin tightening and raising the low and superficial skin-hydration levels. Diminishing the signs of photo aging, like dark spots and broken capillaries, helps representatives of the sagging type look younger.

As sagging skin has lower levels of hydration, it takes a longer time to repair skin elasticity. Dehydrated skin is not able to respond to the treatment as efficiently as hydrated skin. That is why I recommend preparation for such serious treatments as laser treatments, skin tightening, and injections. The goal for such a preparation is to build the hydration reserve of the skin. Only moisturized skin responds to serious stimulation like skin tightening. Sagging skin will get lots of benefits from skin tightening (the treatment of choice) as well as fillers and volumizing injections.

Types of Aging: Tired

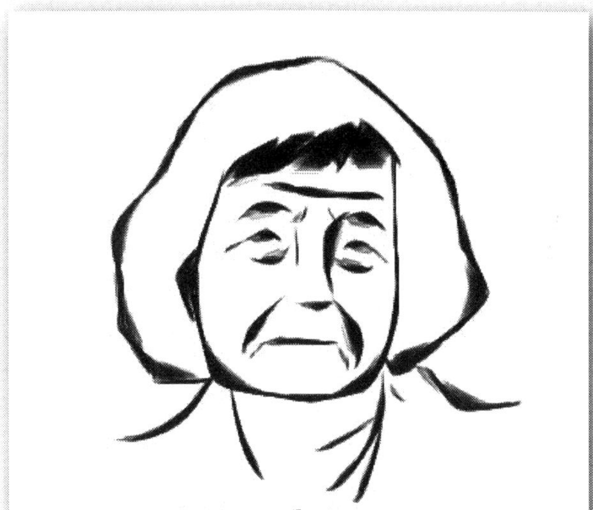
Tired type

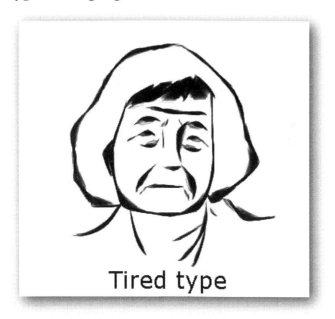

People with this type of aging have complaints about their faces getting swollen from their twenties. Coworkers and relatives point out to members of this type that some days they do not look good because of the signs of fatigue on their faces.

People with this type of aging are usually not overweight. The shape of their faces resembles an oval or a rhombus. The first signs of this type of aging appear with droopy eyelids, depressed eye angles, and nasolabial folds.

It usually happens in the late thirties. These people complain of decreasing tone and elasticity after forty. Very often, they see facial asymmetry as a result of the muscle imbalance. Their jaws show aging after fifty when the facial-fat repositioning process is started.

Representatives of the tired aging type do not have as good lymphatic-drainage function and capillary flow as people of other types do. That explains the appearance of deep wrinkles, folds, and jowls. The skin is well-moisturized during youth and becomes drier with age.

Treatment Plan for the Tired Type

Any type of treatment that has the goal of improving lymphatic drainage and microcirculation will be beneficial for the tired type. The next goal is increasing skin elasticity through the skin-tightening process.

For restoration of skin elasticity, there are two technologies: laser and RF technology.

Both stimulate the collagen- and elastin-formation processes. Laser does it through injury, whereas RF employs *raising* the temperature in the deeper skin layers. There is also a new technology called *fractional RF*. This technology stimulates collagen and elastin growth by damaging the skin through thermal-zone injuries and heating the deep skin layers simultaneously. These systems work for skin tightening and increasing skin elasticity.

Despite the fact that the tired type of aging does not require as much fat removal as the deformative type does, some fat deposits demand correction, especially in the lower one-third of the face. Fat removal is quite a complicated process in itself. The marketing stories about creams and masks that help get rid of double chins are not accurate. These areas are too deep to be reached with any type of cream or mask; it should be done with technology.

To remove fat, there are two processes: the adipocyte (fat cell) death process and lymphatic drainage. The target is to kill fat cells and remove the products of metabolism from the area.

The best technology for killing fat cells, from my practical view, is radiofrequency (RF) technology. A combination of RF and vacuum mechanical massage in one treatment will be more effective. Vacuum mechanical massage helps to stimulate lymphatic drainage too. Specialists should consider working with tired skin types simultaneously with different technologies, targeting skin tightening, lymphatic drainage, and fat removal in one treatment session. Such an approach guarantees the results of skin tightening, eye lifting, wrinkle diminishing, and facial contouring. An additional touch of neurotoxin in the upper one-third of the face and filler injections is able to remove ten years from the appearance.

Types of Aging: Deformative

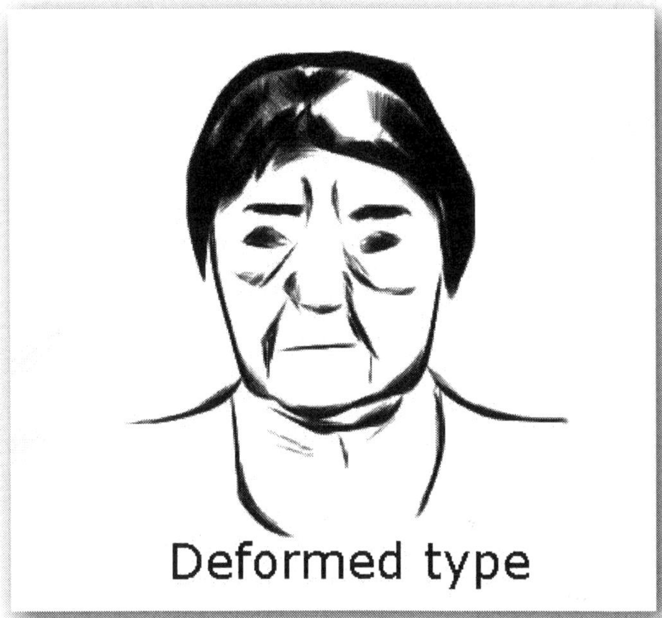

People prone to being overweight are predisposed to this type of aging. Usually, people of this group do not have wrinkles. The main sign of aging is gravitational *ptosis*. Ptosis is a result of redeposition of the fat. Redeposition of the fat from the middle one-third to the lower one-third of the face makes the jawline almost invisible, and a double chin replaces this line.

The appearance of a double chin and the deformation of the facial shape occur because of the fat-dropping process. It impacts the middle and the lower thirds of the face and the general area of the neck. The skin stretches out because of the pressure from the fat and as the result of aging itself.

Also, people with the deformative type of aging often have damaged microcirculation and insufficient lymphatic drainage. This means that they are prone to keeping the liquid in the interstitial space, which makes this area of the face even heavier.

Other signs such as droopy cheeks and eyelids, a wavy jawline, jowls, fat pockets in the area of the lower eyelids, and nasolabial folds are typical indicators of the deformative type of aging.

Treatment Plan for the Deformative Type

The treatment plan for this type of aging should include fat removal, shrinking the skin layers, skin tightening, and improving the lymphatic drainage as well as microcirculation.

The first two or three treatments should have the goal of fat removal from the lower one-third of the face and from the neck area. Lymphatic drainage in this case should be considered as the pathway for removing the broken fat cells. A combination of RF and vacuum technologies results in impressive changes after three or four treatments. The delivery of lipolytic substances into the deep skin layers with needles or without them works well for the fat-removal process.

After fat removal, the goal of treatment shifts to the process of skin tightening and shrinking the skin layers. From my personal experience, the combination of radiofrequency technology (RF) and fractional RF works the best.

Additional deep skin hydration should be included in the treatment plan of the skin after the age of forty.

Clients should be prepared to wait a period of time no less than two months to see any significant changes in the shape of the face if they make the choice of nonsurgical correction.

Types of Aging: Muscular

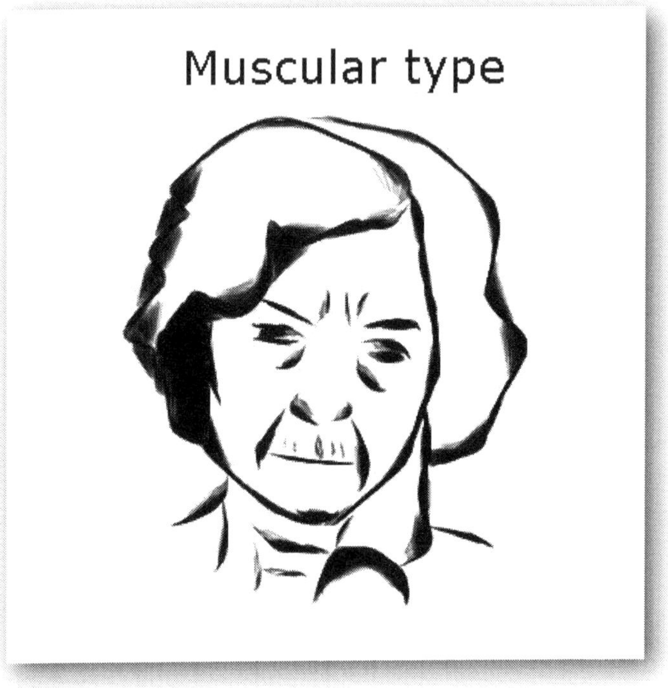

Mostly people of Asian descent have this type of aging. In the muscular type of aging, the muscles of the face are very strong. Wrinkles and folds in the areas of the upper and lower eyelids and nasolabial folds appear as signs of aging, as well as drooping corners of the lips. The skin texture remains smooth, barely showing signs of sagginess, and the face keeps its shape up to the senior years. Most of the people who age with the muscular skin type see dark spots and discoloration on their faces in their early forties.

Treatment Plan for the Muscular Type

The main goal is releasing the muscle spasm in the lower one-third of the face. Injections of neurotoxins work to release the muscle tension and make the jawline smoother. If the client refuses to do injections, any type of massage will work with the same goal. A combination of technologies for the superficial skin layer helps to remove dark spots.

Types of Aging: Combination of Types

This type includes all the previous signs. The treatment plan should involve fat removal, reparation of the skin's elasticity and tone, and restoration of the microcirculation and lymphatic drainage.

Scientists in the world endlessly discuss different theories of the aging process, but the main point remains the same: it is impossible to avoid completely something that has been genetically programmed.

In the twenty-first century, we prolong youth. We do it using the technological progress the humankind has made. A combination of technologies is not only able to obtain an aesthetic result but also able to influence the mechanisms the aging process is based on. Influencing these mechanisms has a therapeutic effect that brings fast, long-term, and safe results.

CHAPTER 3

Gravity - Droopy Eyelids, Nasolabial Folds, Jowls, Double Chins

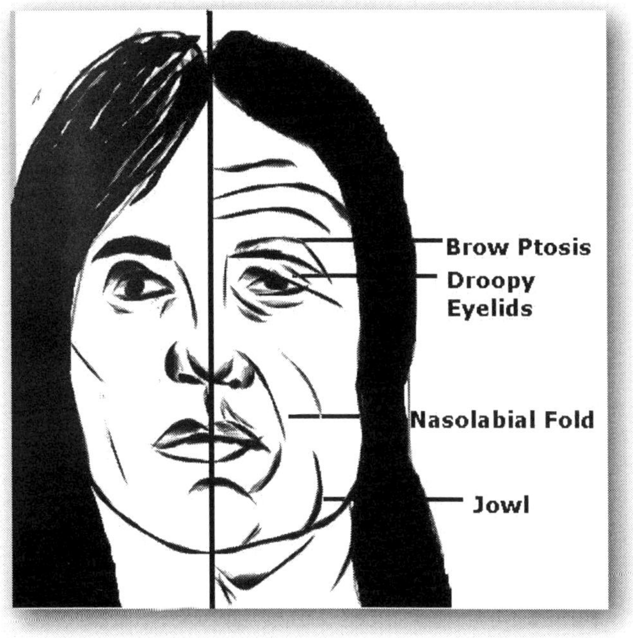

When droopy eyelids, nasolabial folds, jowls, or double chins appear, we rarely blame gravity. We say, "I did not sleep well," "It's stress," or "I worked too much." But after forty, it is gravity. Droopy eyelids, bags under the eyes, tear-throughs, nasolabial folds, unclear face contouring, and double chins are all signs of gravity affecting us.

There are three stages of gravity effects on the face.

Gravity: First Stage

It starts with the upper part of the face. When we are young, we have the perfect shape of eyebrows—wavy, not horizontal. When the outer parts of the eyebrows shift horizontally, it is time to ring the bell. Aging has started.

Creases are visible in the upper eyelids when the eyes are open. These creases do not touch the eyelash edge, and they disappear when the eyes close. Dark circles under the eyes attract attention. Dark circles are the result of visible blood vessels. The explanation for such changes is simple. It is the process of the destruction of the eye orbit and muscle weakness. The first lines, called nasolacrimal and nasolabial lines, draw our attention in the mirror. Some clients see bags under their eyes, which disappear when they smile.

What is the reason for first-stage gravity changes?
The first-stage gravity changes are mostly on the level of imperfect lymphatic drainage and microcirculation. In some areas, the process of replacing cross-linked collagen with new collagen is slower. It is the exact reason for the visibility of lines. Skin dehydration plays a role in the appearance of signs of the first-stage gravity as well.

Treatment Plan for First-Stage Gravity Changes

Lymphatic drainage can improve the condition of first-stage gravity changes. No less than ten treatments will be required. Treatment is more effective with faster results when systems for lymphatic drainage are used.

Skin tightening or laser treatments in the areas of concern help to stimulate new collagen production and microcirculation. Mesotherapy with a needle or needle-free aids in the hydration of the superficial and deep skin layers by creating a depot of active substances inside the skin. Filler and neurotoxin injections also work very well to hydrate and lift up the tissue.

Gravity: Second Stage

When wrinkles on the nose bridge become visible, it is time to pay precise attention to the gravity process. Droopy eyelids and crow's-feet are two symptoms people want to get rid of the most.

Droopy eyelids occur when creases of the upper eyelid lie on the eyelashes, regardless of whether the eyes are open or closed. The outer and inner angles of the eyes are on the same line (normally the outer should be three to five millimeters higher). Repositioning of fat in the middle part of the face is a reason for the appearance of tear-throughs and nasolabial folds. The middle part of the face shows significant drooping at the corners of the mouth and increasing in-depth marionette lines. The lower third of the face is marked with the jawline, which is not clear anymore. Jowls interrupt this line. Decreasing the tone of the tissue under the chin area shows up as a double chin or turkey neck.

What Is the Reason for Second-Stage Gravity Changes?

Changes in the depths of muscles, bones, and skin, including the collagen layer, blood vessels, and lymphatic vessels, reflect the aging process called the second stage of gravity.

Treatment Plan for Second-Stage Gravity Changes

The second stage of gravity demands much more comprehensive correction compared with the first stage.

The total correction category of treatment of the face and neck will be required. Skin-tightening RF, fat removal, and laser treatments are all there to help but give results only when they are combined. It is possible to rely only on this series of treatment but not single, sporadic procedures.

Local correction treatments (neurotoxin, fillers, volumizers, and threads) might only be considered as follow-up treatment to the total correction program. Some kinds of injections or fillers based on hyaluronic acid might not correct the gravitational ptosis of stage 2 and might even make it worse.

People with swollen and deformative types of aging experience problems in their lymphatic systems and with lymphatic drainage. Hyaluronic acid (HA) is the base of many fillers, and it is a substance that supports local water retention in tissues. After some kinds of HA injections, the face receives additional volume, but it is the volume of edema. The result of this temporary volume might be additional ptosis of tissues and potential fibrosis in the future.

Gravity: Third Stage (Fifty-Plus Years)

The aggravation of the appearance of gravitational ptosis is expected in the third stage. Such skin changes as skin thinning, shortening and thinning of the red line of the lips, replacing wrinkles with folds, and flattening of the bones are signs of the third stage of gravity.

Treatment Plan for Third-Stage Gravity Changes

Such treatments as facials with deep cleaning, masks, and massages do not bring satisfaction to clients anymore.

It becomes clear that treatments should stimulate processes deep within the skin. Lasers, fractional RF, RF skin tightening, deep chemical peels, and mesotherapy (needle or needle-free) are able to work in such depths.

Unfortunately, an immediate result after the treatment would be a miracle. In most cases, a result can be expected two months after the program has started. Two months is the time for the new collagen-formation process to be visible.

Neurotoxins, fillers, and threads become must-haves in addition to the total correction plan.

If the results of nonsurgical treatments do not satisfy a client, surgery is another option to achieve the desired outcome.

The earlier you start, the longer you will keep the appearance of youth. All three stages of gravity are corrected perfectly when the goal to look younger is based on a comprehensive approach to getting results.

Postmenopausal women should remember that a program of treatments works better than episodic treatments, even quite expensive ones.

Individual treatment protocol with scheduled treatments of one or two times per month will keep you looking younger for many years, whereas sporadic treatments will not.

The kind of program that will be selected and offered to keep you looking younger is the responsibility of your aesthetic specialist, but it is possible to look ten years younger nowadays using new aesthetic-medicine achievements!

CHAPTER 4

Eyes–Wrinkles, Puffiness, and Darkness under the Eyes

Injections, surgeries, and technologies mislead us in the perception of age, but we know quite well what a young face is. A young face shows an active expression, wide-open eyes (even without makeup), round and lifted cheeks, bright skin color, and only a few wrinkles. When time flies, as we also know it does, the face starts to change. What are the real signs of aging? And why does Mother Nature make us look older? Understanding the process makes it easier to battle with aging successfully.

A New Look at the Aging Process

Wrinkles and folds are natural signs of aging. Years ago, we used to think that face wrinkles and folds were the result of insufficient collagen formation and skin dehydration. Today, we look at this problem more closely.

Besides including collagen and elastin production, we also list the following as part of our aging process: bone-structure changes, muscle-spasm processes, microcirculation, and lymphatic drainage as well as all levels of hydration.

If the tone of the muscles increases, the muscles get shorter. This muscle shortness blocks the lymphatic flow and, as a result, contributes to the accumulation of excess fluid. This residual fluid is the cause of the tissue swelling. Swollen tissue is one of the reasons for impaired microcirculation. Bad circulation means that tissues are not supplied with nutrients and oxygen as they should be. New collagen- and elastin-generation processes suffer, as does skin hydration.

If the swelling process is prolonged over time or if it is remittent, fluids and waste products accumulate in the area. The result is tissue swelling, followed by tissue sclerosis, and then tissue fibrosis. Such is the complicated mechanism of tissue aging.

Eyes and the Upper One-Third of the Face—How It Starts

The correction of the aging process in the upper third of the face is very important if one wants to look younger. Crow's-feet, frown lines, and horizontal forehead wrinkles may all alter the appearance of the face. Even insignificant changes in the forehead area, eyebrow line, and periorbital area can be accepted by other people as signs of age subconsciously.

Aging begins somewhere between the ages of eighteen and twenty-eight in the upper part of the face. The first signs are dynamic wrinkles—marks of emotional expression. Later, these wrinkles around the eyes, known as crow's-feet, do not disappear, even when the muscles are relaxed. Impaired collagen-formation processes and skin dehydration play significant roles in such wrinkles' appearance.

For some people, the first sign of aging is *puffy eyelids* or even a puffy face. Usually puffiness is most noticeable in the morning after a sleepless night or after a heavy dinner with a lot of alcohol or salty food. Later, clients mention puffiness as a stable condition that is not correlated with the alleviation of the mentioned factors. Mostly lymphatic stasis determines such a condition.

Eyes That Show Aging

Between forty and fifty, aging begins to affect the upper parts of the face more. Puffy eyelids, dark circles, sagging skin around the eyes, shallow and deep wrinkles, and droopy eyelids are marks that show one's age.

Puffy Eyelids

Puffy eyelids are a sign of aging. It is the aggravation of the process started earlier in age. There are two reasons for puffy eyelids after forty:

hernia and swollen tissue. Hernia is a weakness of thin and stretched-out connective tissues, which should hold fat in the area of the lower eyelid. Tissue swelling is a lymphatic-drainage problem. If the process of tissue swelling is permanent, the skin in the area of the lower eyelid loses its elasticity and stretches out. Squeezing the eyes and being overly expressive are more reasons for fluids to stack up in the periorbital area.

There are two recommended ways of diagnosing hernia versus tissue swelling.

1. Hernia disappears in a horizontal position, but swelling does not.
2. Hernia doesn't change during the day, whereas swelling decreases.

There are several reasons for puffy eyelids:

1. Genetic predisposition that correlates with anatomy, microcirculation, fat tissue, and connective-tissue structures

2. Placing one's face into the pillow during sleep
3. Salty foods and alcohol consumption before bedtime
4. A low-protein diet
5. Unprotected exposure to the sun

How to Get Rid of Puffy Eyelids

Tissue swelling can be removed using vacuum massage. A microdermabrasion system might be a good tool to help with puffiness under the eyes as well.

Heat applied in the area under the eyes promotes the growth of new capillaries. Improved microcirculation helps the area to get rid of excessive fluids. RF technology is used with such a goal.

Surgery is one of the options for treating hernia. Another option is skin tightening that helps the hernia to be less visible.

Dark Circles

Dark circles might show hyperpigmentation or dark spots under the eyes. When the skin under the eyes is thin, sometimes the veins look through the eyes like dark circles. Shadows may appear in the hollows underneath the eyes because of the underlying bone structure changing as the result of the aging process.

How to Get Rid of Dark Circles under the Eyes

- If dark circles under the eyes are the result of hyperpigmentation, the treatment plan includes treatments to destroy this pigmentation. Superficial pigment is removed by microdermabrasion or chemical peel. Darker skin types demand specific chemical peels that include starting the peel in a clinic and home-care products that continuously stimulate skin layers to turn over in two months or more. Effective treatments based on chemical peels produce an unpleasant burning sensation on the treated area throughout this two-month period.
- If dark circles under the eyes are the result of thin skin and vein shadows, a

skin-tightening eye-lift program will be the best solution.

Eye Lines—Sagging Skin with Lots of Shallow or Deep Wrinkles

There are some reasons for wrinkles around the eyes. Treatment is based on the particular reason.

- If undereye lines are the result of skin dehydration in the area around the eyes, hyaluronic-acid injections or needle-free delivery into the superficial and deep layers of the skin will be the best solution.
- If the reason is the hyperfunction of muscles, we use neurotoxin injections. It takes about ten to twelve units of the substance to get an optimal result, which can be maintained by reinjecting this area every three months.
- If the reason for the lines under the eyes is decreasing skin elasticity, RF eye-lift skin tightening is the treatment of choice.

Radiofrequency (RF) penetrates into the layer of collagen, elastin, and hyaluronic acid, which stimulates growth. In order to achieve an excellent result, the RF energy is delivered directly to the skin collagen layer.

Asymmetrically Dropped Eyebrows

Asymmetry is a sign of the aging process that in most cases should be corrected with RF skin tightening, at least six treatments, followed by neurotoxin injections.

To Get Rid of Droopy Eyelids

To get rid of droopy eyelids, it is necessary to shrink the skin layer in the upper-eyelid area. The process of shrinking the skin is called skin tightening. Skin-tightening treatment is based on RF technology. Droopy-eyelid treatment with RF technology is based on the science of RF. Heating the deep skin layer up to 43°C immediately destroys damaged collagen cross-links and stimulates the production of new collagen. We shrink and tighten the layer of sagging skin in the upper eyelid.

Peptides and hyaluronic acid should be delivered into the skin immediately after the RF treatment. Delivery might be done with needle or needle-free mesotherapy. Peptides and hyaluronic acid work as a collagen booster to stimulate new collagen synthesis, getting rid of the droopy eyelids.

How to Conceal the Signs of Aging under the Eyes

Aesthetic medicine is able to successfully conceal these signs of aging. Injections of fillers and neurotoxin, combined with RF skin tightening, give the desired result.

RF skin tightening changes the skin's condition and stimulates new collagen formation, when the neurotoxin assumes the role of a local corrector, soothing muscles. Combining these technologies with skin hydration (needle or needle-free mesotherapy), we achieve quick results with a high level of client satisfaction.

The right diagnosis is based on the understanding that the key to successful treatment of aging around the eyes is the universal statement made throughout my entire book that each treatment demands a thoughtful approach for every client.

CHAPTER 5

Acne—A Comprehensive Approach for Fast Results

Acne is a disease. Hypersensitivity to the male hormones plays a key role in the onset of acne. The mechanism of acne is complicated enough. We can only guess what the main factor in the appearance of acne is, but we never know why some people get acne and others don't. To understand what happens and how we get pimples, we will talk about the causes of acne we know about.

The following are some factors that predispose one to acne:

1. A lot of dead cells on the top skin layer
2. A high level of oil production by sebaceous glands

3. Microcomedones—what you feel under the fingers
4. The growth of bacteria inside of the clogged sebaceous glands

The first factor is an abnormal number of dead cells in the top skin layer. The dead cells clog the sebaceous glands, forming a plug. Closed sebaceous glands create a nourishing environment for bacterial growth. The second factor is increased sebum production. The third factor pertains to the inflammation of the follicles that produce microcomedones, commonly referred to as a *blackhead* (containing an opening to the skin surface).

Enlarged microcomedones that don't open to the skin surface are called *whiteheads*. It's quite common for clients not to be able to see them but to be able to feel them when touching the skin with fingers. Stretching out the skin allows whiteheads to become visible. *They are inflamed under the stream of hormonal disturbances and show up on the skin as pimples.*

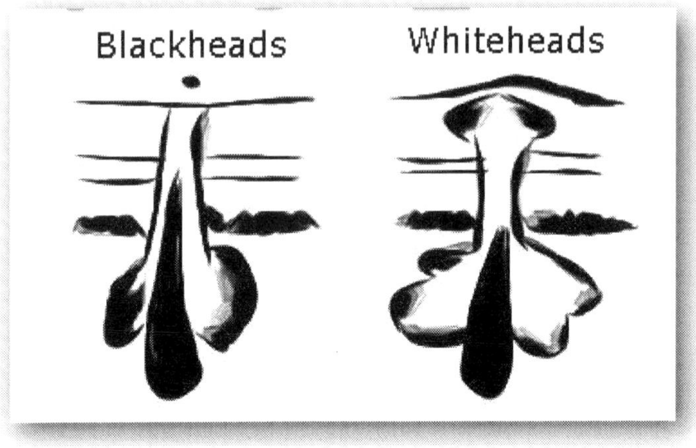

The last factor for acne onset is bacterial growth. Clogged sebaceous glands encourage the growth of bacteria in the oil-rich environment. This proliferation stimulates inflammation. Inflammation results in pimple growth.

There are three levels of acne severity: mild, moderate, and severe.

Mild acne generally consists of noninflammatory and inflammatory acne lesions, which could be simultaneously open or closed comedones.

Moderate acne includes more extensive comedonal acne or papules and pustules.

Severe acne appears as nodules and cysts, causes scarring, and coexists with comedonal and papulopustular lesions.

Success in Acne Treatment

To be successful in acne treatment, it is a necessity to influence all the mechanisms that trigger its appearance.

1. Normalize the process of skin turnover.
2. Normalize the production of sebum.
3. Take control of the emergence of the microcomedones.
4. End the growth of the bacteria.
5. Raise the skin's overall immunity.

Ways to Treat Acne

There are three ways to treat acne: medical-spa treatments, topical treatments, and systemic treatments using medications.

Before choosing a treatment plan, it is necessary to diagnose the leading causes of the acne.

You might choose medical-spa treatments with cosmeceutical-grade care products, medical-spa treatments with topical or systemic medications, or even all of them together. The choice should be made with the assistance of a treatment provider.

Choose the Right Treatment for You

The natural way to handle acne is medical-spa treatments. There are various types of them, including microdermabrasion, chemical peels, IPL photofacials, radiofrequency skin tightening, and mesotherapy. These treatments are highly effective and the least harmful because of the lack of systemic influence and the lowest risk of side effects.

A combination of technologies achieves better and more long-lasting results. A combination of technologies shows improvement in the acne after the first or second procedure in the cases of mild to moderate acne.

If three to five treatments don't result in impressive outcomes, topical medications should be added. If the combination of medical-spa treatments and topical medications don't accomplish the desired effect, I advise adding systemic medications. And if even this course of treatment does not achieve the desired results, I suggest using retinoids, but there are numerous side effects that need to be kept in mind.

Medical-Spa Acne Treatment

Diamond Microdermabrasion

Microdermabrasion is used to remove dead cells from the top skin layer and normalize oil production. Dead-cell removal curbs the risk of clogging the sebaceous glands. In addition, their regular turnover improves the skin's hydration. Skin hydration increases the skin's immunity.

Chemical Peels

Use of the chemical peels depends entirely on the case of acne and the condition of the patient's skin. The following is a list of peels used in acne treatment:

- Azelaic peel
- Salicylic peel
- Mindalic peel
- Glycolic peel
- Jessner peel
- Retinol peel

Just like microdermabrasion, the chemical peels are used for dead-cell turnover. Some also regulate oil production by the sebaceous glands. Some have antibacterial and anti-inflammatory effects.

The right chemical peel should be chosen by the treatment provider after comprehensive assessment of the client. Such a choice is based on the main triggering mechanism of the acne.

IPL Photofacial (Intense Pulsed Light)

A special laser has been developed for acne treatment. The intense pulsed light (IPL) photofacial uses light to trigger the pigment inside the closed sebaceous glands and destroy the bacteria. The result is normalizing the production of excess sebum and decreasing the inflammation. Combined efforts significantly lower the frequency of breakouts.

IPL provides noncoherent pulses of visible light (having longer wavelengths than blue light). IPL is able to penetrate deeper into the follicle to suppress the bacterial growth and to stimulate the healing process.

Radiofrequency Skin Tightening for Acne Treatment

Whereas RF was designed to improve skin laxity, it has recently been studied in the treatment of inflammatory acne. High temperatures kill bacteria and shrink sebaceous glands.

Fractional Radiofrequency is widely used for acne-scar treatment with results after the first procedure.

Skin Hydration

To force the healing process and raise immunity, *needle-free mesotherapy* or *traditional mesotherapy* is used. In cases where the skin is dry and it demands additional hydration, hyaluronic acid helps.

Hyaluronic acid not only increases the skin's hydration but also normalizes the skin's pH level. Skin immunity depends on skin pH. High immunity prevents the inflammation of the microcomedones. Well-hydrated skin forces the healing process too.

Topical Acne Treatment

Topical acne treatments target mild to moderate acne, which includes inflammatory and noninflammatory forms. Retinoids (tretinoin, adapalene, and tazarotene) influence on the process of exfoliation and interfere with the microcomedone formation. Topical retinoids alone are indicative of noninflammatory acne.

Adapalene is a less-irritating alternative to topical tretinoin. A second-line retinoid is tazarotene, which is a teratogeic. It is prohibited for use in women of child-bearing potential.

Benzoyl peroxide, a topical bactericidal agent, works as an inhibitor of *bacteria*. Of note, benzoyl peroxide does not induce bacterial resistance.

Topical antibiotics alone are also effective treatments of acne, but just like the systemic antibiotics, they are associated with resistance.

Azelaic acid works very well in removing the superficial layer of dead cells and as an antibacterial agent. Azelaic acid is available in a variety of creams and gels.

Systemic-Acne Treatment

Systemic Antibiotics

Systemic antibiotics are recommended for moderate to severe acne and are prescribed for treatment-resistant forms of inflammatory acne. The most commonly prescribed antibiotics for acne are tetracycline, erythromycin, clindamycin, doxycycline, and minocycline.

Before using oral antibiotics, remember that they are associated with gastrointestinal irritation and vaginal candidiasis.

Hormonal Agents

Hormonal therapy reduces sebum production caused by androgenic overstimulation and decreases the androgen responsiveness of sebaceous glands. Hormonal agents, such as estrogen-containing oral contraceptives and the oral antiandrogens spironolactone and cyproterone acetate, are used.

Corticosteroid Therapy

Short-term and low-dose oral corticosteroid therapy may provide temporary benefits for severe inflammatory acne.

Isotretinoin

Isotretinoin is prescribed for use for cases of severe acne or for treatment-resistant acne, resulting in physical scarring.

Isotretinoin is the only systemic agent that has anti-inflammatory action, inhibits sebum production, and shrinks the sebaceous glands.

Clients taking isotretinoin have been reported to experience mood disorders, depression, suicidal ideation, and suicide attempts.

Isotretinoin is a teratogen. Female patients of child-bearing potential may be treated with isotretinoin only with some conditions.

Food and Acne

Chocolate is rich in biologically active compounds (caffeine, theobromine, and serotonin), which increase secretion of insulin and its peripheral resistance. Chocolate has an effect on the processes involved in the occurrence of acne lesions. Certain individuals consuming chocolate may be exposed to more frequent incidents or worsening of acne lesions.

Milk consumption too has been linked to acne because milk is an insulinotropic nutrient that increases serum insulin levels. Some studies reported a connection between frequent milk consumption and acne severity.

Skimmed-milk intake causes a breakout or worsening of acne too. However, yogurt consumption is not correlated with acne occurrence.

Lactoferrin-enriched fermented milk decreases acne severity, owing to the anti-inflammatory effects of lactoferrin and its ability to suppress microbial growth. An intake of polyunsaturated fatty acids (omega-6 and omega-3) modulates the skin's inflammatory responses. Intake of omega-3 fatty acids may contribute to a decrease in acne.

Eight Simple Tips to Protect Your Skin from Breakouts

1. Do not mess with your pimples and blemishes yourself! This can spread bacteria and make acne worse.
2. Everyday rule—change your pillowcases.
3. Everyday rule—clean your cell phone with alcohol or hand sanitizer daily.
4. Do not wear makeup at the gym.
5. Before and after hair removal by waxing, tweezing, and depilatories, use hydrocortisone, by applying a thin layer on the skin.
6. Be mindful of stress.
7. Pick the right nonirritating sunscreen.
8. Wash your face! Never sleep with makeup on!

CHAPTER 6

Dark Spots that People Pay Attention to and Melasma

Melasma is a disorder of skin pigmentation. The pigment (melanin) is synthesized by pigment cells (melanocytes). We see the deposit of the melanin (melanin granules) as hyperpigmentation. Pigment spots occur typically later in life and look like light-gray to dark-brown patches. They appear mostly on sun-exposed areas, such as faces and arms.

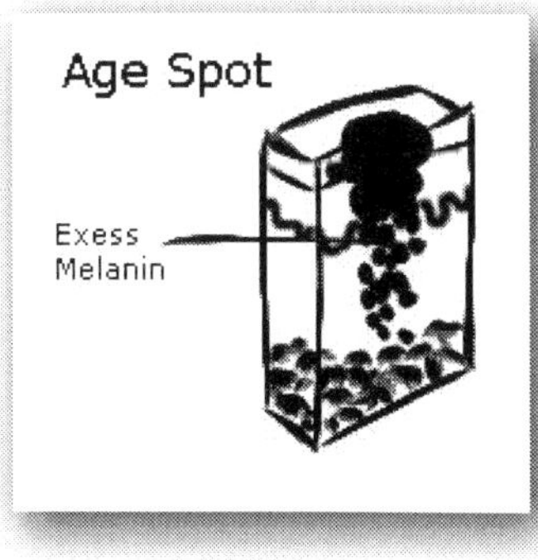

Psychologists insist that subconscious evaluation of age is based on the even color of the skin. The more even the skin tone is, the younger the person looks. Might be it explains the total dependence on makeup? Does that mean that by removing dark spots, it is possible to look ten years younger?

Aesthetic medicine can significantly diminish all areas of hyperpigmentation, but it is impossible to completely remove some of them, especially melasma areas. The result of the battle with melasma depends on how deeply it has localized. To understand the depth, we use Wood's lamp. Using Wood's lamp, we can see the superficial hyperpigmentation, called epidermal melasma, but not melasma that has spread deeper into the skin.

Epidermal melasma is the most common type of melasma; melanin is found in all epidermal (superficial skin) layers. Patients with epidermal melasma usually show an excellent response to the therapy.

- Dermal melasma is a skin condition in which pigment cells are found throughout the entire dermis (deep skin layer). The pigmentation is not visible under Wood's lamp examination. Patients with dermal melasma show a poor response to therapy.

- A mixed type is when pigment cells are found in both layers: epidermis and dermis. During Wood's lamp examination, there is an intensification of melanin in some areas, while in others, there is attenuation or no change. Patients with mixed type show good response to therapy too.

Patients with darker skin type have indeterminate melasma, and there are no findings with Wood's lamp examination.

It is very easy to understand how the melasma treatment should be planned.

First, in order to treat melasma, it is necessary to remove the pigment from the top skin layer and disrupt the melanin granules. We employ chemical peels and microdermabrasion for the purpose of pigment removal. And for disruption of melanin granules, lasers have given us good results.

In the second step, the objective is inhibition of the activity of the melanocytes (melanocytes are cells responsible for the pigment synthesis). Protection from sunlight and avoidance of precipitating factors, such as ultraviolet (UV) and visible light, are crucial for this purpose. It looks like no stimulation, no skin activity.

And the final step is aimed at the inhibition of the synthesis of melanin (pigment) by the pigment cells. Using bleaching agents is important for this purpose.

As with most individual treatments, it should be tailored to the patient's needs.

Currently, we don't know the factors and reasons behind the emergence of melasma. We attribute it to sunlight and genetic predisposition.

The main risk factor for hyperpigmentation is exposure to natural or artificial UV radiation as well as hormonal factors, which are crucial in the appearance of the melasma. Hormonal disturbances or the intake of oral contraceptives and pregnancy are aggravating factors.

Some cosmetic substances, such as oxidized linoleic acid, salicylate, citral, and preservatives, can be triggering factors for melasma. Medications described as phototoxic or photosensitive, such as anticonvulsants, have been associated with melasma too.

Treatment of dark spots is based on some patterns: Start with microdermabrasion and topical agents. Microdermabrasion is a mechanical peel that removes the superficial dead cells and pigment cells. It is able to mechanically remove superficial hyperpigmentation. Some clients ask if it is possible to experience aggravation of hyperpigmentation after microdermabrasion. The answer is if it is a diamond-microdermabrasion system used by a professional with experienced hands, then the risk is minimal, approximately 0.001 percent.

Sunscreen should be used following the treatment.

Hydroquinone

Hydroquinone (HQ) has been used for over fifty years as a hyperpigmentation treatment. It works by inhibiting the tyrosinase activity (enzyme that's significantly involved in the process of pigment-cell synthesis) and increases the degradation of the cells that produce pigment. Hydroquinone is only active in epidermal (superficial) melasma; it is inactive in the dermal layer of the skin. The use of 3–5 percent HQ is recommended for melasma, while lower concentrations of 2 percent are used as a maintenance therapy.

The most common side effect of HQ is irritant or allergic contact dermatitis. It is associated with dosage, concentration, and duration of application.

Permanent gray-brown or blue-black hyperpigmentation with pinpoint, dark-brown (caviar-like) patches usually result from prolonged application of high-concentration HQ. This condition is called exogenous ochronosis and is the most serious side effect of HQ treatment.

In the European Union, HQ has been banned from use as a cosmetic ingredient since 2001 for concerns about ochronosis and occupational vitiligo.

Kojic Acid

Kojic acid is an effective nonprescription bleaching agent. It is a product of fungal metabolism. Kojic acid inhibits tyrosinase (enzyme) activity. Side effects include sensitivity and allergic contact dermatitis. Kojic acid may be used alone at a concentration of 1–4 percent twice daily or together with other acids.

Azelaic Acid

Azelaic acid works by inhibiting tyrosinase (enzyme) and affecting hyperactive melanocytes (cells that produce melanin pigment) without affecting the ordinary melanocytes. Azalaic acid works as an anti-inflammatory agent too. It is an over-the-counter treatment for melasma.

Azalaic acid is recommended for use twice daily for three or more months. It is a very well-accepted topical antihyperpigmentation agent.

Tretinoin

Tretinoin is a retinoic acid and is the most commonly used topical retinoid for the treatment of melasma. It acts by halting the melanin-stimulating superficial cells' turnover process. Tretinoin is recommended at a concentration of 0.01–0.1 percent, and better results are obtained when used in a combination formula with HQ.

Combination Formula

For increasing efficacy (skin bleaching), minimizing side effects, and decreasing the duration of the treatment period, a combination formula is used. The triple combination formula of HQ, retinoid, and corticosteroid leads to even better results, as the three ingredients jointly act in enhancing the effect. The formula is also better accepted by clients. The best-known triple combination formula of HQ, tretinoin, and topical corticosteroid is the Kligman-Willis formula. An application for five to seven weeks is recommended with this treatment.

IPL Photofacial

More aggressive treatments have the risk of postinflammatory hyperpigmentation (PIH). Bleaching agents prepare the skin for more aggressive treatment, greatly diminishing the side effects of IPL treatment. Side effects of this therapy are minimal and usually include a burning sensation during treatment and redness some hours after. The success of IPL treatment is higher in clients with superficial hyperpigmentation.

Fractional Systems

Nonfractional lasers are not as popular as they were years ago for the treatment of melasma. Compared with nonfractional laser, fractional systems go through the skin like pixel cameras, injuring the skin in some areas but leaving the skin between these thermal zones intact. This technique helps the skin to recover much faster without the risk of a postinflammatory hyperpigmentation (PIH).

Fractional lasers, such as fractional RF (fractional radiofrequency) systems, are the treatment of choice for the mixed and dermal types of melasma. Some fractional RF treatments work for patients with skin types IV through VI (darker skin types).

Mesotherapy

Mesotherapy offers delivery of the skin-active ingredients that are able to block tyrosinase (enzyme). Delivered substances, such as kojic acid, vitamin C, and arbutin, work in the direction of blocking tyrosinase 9 (enzyme) and preventing postinflammatory hyperpigmentation, especially after IPL, fractional RF, or laser treatments.

There are two types of mesotherapy on the market: needle mesotherapy and needle-free (electroporation) mesotherapy. Using needles might be a trigger for an aggravation of hyperpigmentation due to the factor of mechanical (needle) trauma. Needle-free mesotherapy offers the delivery of substances without the risk of PIH.

As there is no clear understanding of why melasma occurs, aesthetic medicine isn't able to give an absolute solution to removing it. Every treatment should be tailored to the individual patient after assessing the depth of his or her pigments.

We use different techniques, technologies, and approaches to target hyperpigmentation at different depths. The combination of IPL, fractional systems, microdermabrasion, chemical peels, and needle-free mesotherapy as well as topical bleaching agents, is proven to provide successful and much better results than monotherapy.

Maintenance therapy should be used for optimal results.

Sunscreen is a must to prevent the aggravation of melasma.

CHAPTER 7

Rosacea

Rosacea is characterized by flushes, redness, and pimples that cover areas of broken capillaries.

We still do not know exactly what the origin of rosacea is. Most experts agree that the disorder is related to blood vessels in the deep skin layer. Under certain stimuli, vessels stay dilated. Permanently dilated vessels provoke the body's response. The body sends immune and inflammatory cells to the area. These cells contribute to the permanent redness and pimples seen.

There are two major components of rosacea: redness and inflammation.

From the beginning, rosacea appears as visible blood vessels on the face (very often around the nose). Within a short time after sun exposure or some food consumption, clients have sensations of stinging and burning. Over the years, persistent redness and flushing show rosacea is progressing. Red pimples on the face reflect the stage of inflammation.

Types of Rosacea

Rosacea can just be a central facial redness. It can be associated with symptoms such as itching, burning, and stinging too.

In addition to redness, some clients develop pimples that tend to fluctuate over time.

There is also the type of rosacea in which the individual develops a bulbous nose. This occurrence is more typical in men than in women.

Swollen and read eyes are one more type of rosacea.

Rosacea Treatment

Rosacea treatment should be focused on removing broken capillaries and stopping the process of inflammation. Raising the skin's immunity is a goal of treatment to prevent rosacea occurrence.

To Get Rid of Rosacea

Patients need to understand that we've come a long way in treating rosacea. At least five treatments will be recommended. The good news is that the results are visible after the first treatment.

It starts with the technology to destroy broken capillaries, so new healthy capillaries will grow. Stopping the inflammation process is the next goal.

When these two goals are accomplished, the skin's even color will be returned. Deep levels of skin hydration will help to raise skin immunity and prevent rosacea's return. Because the reason for rosacea's appearance is not clear, a comprehensive approach to treating rosacea is obvious.

I would suggest including several technologies in every rosacea treatment, starting with very gentle microdermabrasion and very soft lymphatic-drainage massage to stimulate the superficial skin cells to grow. New cells have higher immunity levels and are better hydrated. To destroy broken capillaries, stop inflammation, and make the skin tone even, IPL (intense pulsed light) photofacials work. To deliver substances that moisturize skin deep into it, needle-free mesotherapy is used. Lasers are a good solution for broken capillary removal.

Some chemical peels give very good results for the treatment of rosacea. Retinol and azelaic peels are the leaders among them. Most clients who have rosacea with pimples declare a 50 percent improvement after one retinol peel. Azelaic acid is a very popular product for home care.

Rosacea Flare Factors

Flare factors aren't consistent for everyone. Hot liquids and hot foods can be flare factors. Spicy food in some cases provokes redness too. Many people blame wine for making their face red. Sun exposure enhances rosacea. For some ethnic groups, the sauna is a trigger. Hot showers and baths should be avoided from the point of common sense. Individuals have to get to know themselves and know what their own flare factors are, and then they can avoid them.

Rosacea Home Care

There are two must-haves in rosacea home care. The first one is hydration. Perfect skin hydration is the key for the skin's immunity. The second is sunscreen, which prevents skin from flaring and becoming inflamed. Other home-care products should not irritate the skin. Scrubs should not be used.

Red faces are very rare among young people. We pay attention to this condition after forty. Then we recall that our parents had red cheeks all their lives. Very often, rosacea is a hereditary condition. But mostly sun and lifestyle are responsible for rosacea. Please pay attention to how the face responds to the sun, to food, and to alcohol. If you see redness, we can help. The earlier you ask us for help, the faster and more permanent will be the result.

CHAPTER 8

The Neck – How to Get Rid of a Double Chin, Circles of the Neck, Cords, and Sagging Skin

One of the major concerns that most women have relates to their necks. This is particularly true of women between the ages of thirty and seventy-five. When I ask my patients, "How do you feel after the neck-lift treatment?" the most common answer I get is, "The way I used to feel when I was way younger." In my experience, women feel happiest when they have a neck lift. The only other thing that even comes close is weight loss.

Different women have different concerns, but all concerns about the neck fall into one of four categories:

1. Double chin
2. Circles of the neck
3. Cords
4. Sagging skin

The good news is effective treatments are available for these conditions.

Double Chin

There are some theoretical issues that explain the reason for the double chin's appearance. We associate double chins with fat drops and shift the responsibility of this dropping to the gravity process. And we are right, but additional mechanisms play a role in this issue. Medically speaking, these processes are triggered not only by fat dropping but also by impaired microcirculation and lymphatic drainage. It is also triggered by weakness of the collagen support.

According to the contemporary view on the problem of double-chin appearance, as the aging process takes place, the muscle in the jaw area shrinks. This shrinkage is the result of muscle hypertension.

Muscle spasms not only destroy the balance of the musculoskeletal structure of the face and neck but also work as an obstacle for the microcirculation and lymphatic (lymph) flow. The result of these processes is the accumulation of the liquid in the lower part of the face and neck. These swollen tissues have the consequences of damaging the microcirculation as well. It is a cycle that needs to and can be broken.

In order to have a tightened skin, our bodies should destroy damaged collagen and produce new. Good microcirculation is one of the key conditions for the restoration process. When circulation is insufficient, the processes of new collagen formation suffer. Fat does not have sufficient collagen support and shows it as jowls.

Double chins are mostly a problem of the deformative type of aging (overweight people very often are representatives of this type). All that was mentioned earlier—microcirculation, lymphatic drainage, and gravity processes with fat dropping and weakness of the collagen support—are conditions for this type of aging. In addition, the deformative type of aging in 40 percent of cases has a hereditary pathology of connective tissues—high levels of immature collagen, which is the reason for decreased amounts of mature collagen and decreased strength of supportive tissues. What this means is that the collagen support of the dropping fat (due to gravity) is not stable and strong compared with that of representatives of other aging types.

Treatment Plan for a Double Chin

Based on such mechanisms, the treatment plan for a double chin is the following:

- Fat removal
- Collagen formation
- Improving the microcirculation
- Improving the lymphatic-drainage function
- Decreasing the spasm of the jaw muscles

Fat Removal and Collagen Stimulation for Double Chins

There are two solutions for fat removal on the aesthetic-medicine market today.

The first is liposuction. Liposuction decreases the number of fat cells, but afterward, we expect worsening of microcirculation and lymphatic drainage. Aging with a double chin is predetermined to have bad circulation and lack of lymphatic flow, so liposuction might be the treatment of choice in a case when it is the only available solution to eliminate the fat. It's also an option when a client insists on the fastest result.

The second way to remove fat from the jaw and neck area is radiofrequency (RF) technology. RF waves raise the temperature in the fat layer of the skin. Scientific research shows that maintaining a temperature of 43°C in the fat layer for ten minutes starts the process of fat cells dying.

However, there is one condition for these treatments to be successful: there should be very good microcirculation in the area of the treatment because the conductive tissue for the RF energy is blood. For blood-circulation improvement, vacuum mechanical massage works the best, and it is confirmed scientifically. Systems that combine vacuuming and RF technology are the most effective. The RF and vacuum technology work together to remove fat and improve the microcirculation and lymph drainage. RF and vacuum technology also release the muscle tension (simply by using deep heat) and stimulate the collagen formation (skin-tightening process). The results emerge immediately after the treatment starts.

Circles of the Neck

Many of my clients say that they had neck circles from early childhood. It's simply true. Neck circles divide fat pockets in the neck area. Due to aging, skin loses its elasticity and tone, making the neck circles become more visible. Circle shadows play a significant role in the appearance of the neck circles too. The shadows appear as the result of getting together pigment and dead cells inside of the circles. Simply speaking, there are lots of dead cells with the pigment cells in the neck circles.

Treatment Plan for Circles of the Neck

1. Restore the skin's elasticity through the collagen-formation process.
2. Treat the circle shadows toward the removal of hyperpigmentation and dead cells.

Collagen Stimulation and Shadows Removal for Circles of the Neck

When I started to work with neck shadows, I tried a lot, including injections, IPL photo treatments, RF skin tightening, and simple microdermabrasion, and never have been satisfied with the result. Two years ago, I tried fractional RF. From my personal professional experience, I reached the conclusion that this treatment gives the fastest and most impressive results with the neck circles. Fractional RF diminishes the circles' appearance through skin tightening and dead-cell and pigment-removal processes.

To stimulate the process of new collagen formation, fractional RF creates thermal-zone injuries outside and heats the tissues deep inside at the same time.

Fractional RF lightens the skin in the areas of circle shadows through the process called medical skin ablation, which looks like dots of burned skin. Fractional RF allows both steps in one treatment: stimulate the process of skin tightening (collagen stimulation deep in the skin) and remove pigment spots that help lighten the circle-shadow areas on the surface.

Cords

Cords are a widespread and common condition of the neck-aging process. People usually see the first signs of cords at the age of forty. Many women and men do not pay attention to them. But they should. It is much easier to prevent cords than to treat them.

Why Do Cords Appear?

As the result of aging, we have a change of the spinal-column structure, hypertension of the muscles, weakness of the collagen-supporting function, and fat depression. All these factors play a role in the occurrence of cords, but the most significant one is changes in a very specific muscle, called platysma.

Platysma is a broad, thin sheet of muscle that rises from the chest and shoulders and passes upward over the clavicles and neck toward the lower face.

As part of aging, the platysma medial fibers attenuate or thicken to create platysmal bands. The situation is aggravated with weak circulation. Weak circulation negatively influences the muscle and also the skin condition. When it shows, it looks like platysmal bands and sagginess of the skin.

Skin on the neck is much less moisturized compared with the face skin. That explains why people with dry skin in the neck area show more significant signs of aging compared with others. For instance, it is proven that Caucasians have lower amounts of the natural moisturizing factor (NMF), which is responsible for deep skin hydration, and show signs of cords in their early fifties.

In addition, many people do not moisturize the superficial skin layer of the neck with creams or masks on a regular basis. That has the consequence of additional dehydration. Decreasing amounts of hyaluronic acid (the "lake" where the cells that produce collagen reside), a sign of aging, also suppresses the moisturizing level of the skin.

Treatment Plan for Cords

The objective of the treatments is to improve the definition of the topographical landmarks of the neck and to tighten the skin on the neck. Cosmetic treatments in the neck typically address the platysma structures and skin.

Improving the circulation in the platysma is the best way to restore it. Better circulation allows the skin to be better supplied with the nutrients and oxygen and prevents the process of occurrence of new cords.

Skin in the neck responds well to skin tightening and hydration treatments.

From my experience, I know that only the combination of technologies and injections is able to make cords much less visible and prevent the deterioration of the situation.

Microcirculation Improvement and Skin Tightening for Cords

Microcirculation restoration should be more aggressive than the usual practice. Fractional RF is able to stimulate the circulation immediately from the top and bottom of the skin, targeting all skin layers in a more aggressive and quicker way. Fractional RF is used for collagen formation too.

The system works by stimulating collagen formation through thermal-zone injuries combined with raising and maintaining heat in the deep skin layer. In order to respond to such an aggressive invasion, the skin should be well hydrated. But quite often, the aging skin, especially in the neck area, suffers from dehydration. That is why for the adequate processing of the old-new collagen exchange, mesotherapy with hyaluronic acid is recommended.

Mesotherapy means injection or needle-free delivery of the hyaluronic acid into deep skin layers. And it is a must-have procedure after any treatment. Such deep hydration helps the skin to respond to any treatment in the proper way.

One more method involves injections of neurotoxins in the cords. It brings some improvement in a three- to six-month period. From my experience, injections of neurotoxins should be done in combination with the fractional RF treatment after three sessions of fractional RF.

Sagging Skin

Often, sagging skin occurs as a mark of aging before cords, circles, or double chins appear. The Caucasian population suffers most from sagging skin on the neck.

Why Are Caucasians Predisposed to Have Sagging Skin?

Here are some explanations:

- Caucasians do not have thick skin in the neck area, when compared with other groups.

- Caucasians have a lesser amount of natural moisturizing factor (less-hydrated skin).
- Because of light skin color, Caucasians show sun damage on the skin faster (sun elastosis).

All these factors influence the appearance of the signs of sagging skin in the neck area between the ages of forty-five and fifty.

Treatment Plan for Sagging Skin

1. Stimulate new collagen formation.
2. Hydrate skin on all levels.

Skin Tightening and Deep Skin Hydration for Sagging Skin

For the treatment of sagging skin in the neck, skin tightening with RF technology has been used for many years, but my experience shows that new fractional RF, combined with the injection or needle-free delivery of hyaluronic acid inside the skin, gives much better results.

Skin tightening using only RF technology shows results in the neck after a series of six to nine treatments. It is quite simple to explain why skin on the neck requires so many treatments to show results. Explanations come from the microcirculation perspective. The conductive tissue for RF technology is blood. Aging microcirculation is not perfect. So, some first treatments with RF will be helpful only to stimulate the microcirculation (we do not use RF with vacuuming that immediately improves circulation on the neck because of skin laxity). Good circulation is a must-have for good results from skin tightening, because blood is a conductive tissue that accumulates heat. Accumulated heat in the layer of collagen, the dermis, stimulates the process of new collagen formation. Collagen formation means skin tightening.

Faster results are possible using more advanced RF technology—fractional RF. Fractional RF works in both directions; it stimulates the cells that produce new collagen in the deep skin layer through heat and creates thermal-zone injuries, which additionally work from the skin surface as collagen stimulators.

Additional deep skin hydration is a must to help the skin on the neck respond in a better way to this treatment. Neck treatments will get benefits from additional hydration with needles (injections of hyaluronic acid or peptides) or using the needle-free technology (e.g., electroporation).

When to Start Nonsurgical Neck Lifts

Noninvasive (nonsurgical) neck lifts should be done when the first signs of aging appear. The longer you wait to get rid of them, the more difficult and expensive the treatment will be. Sometimes even three months' time plays a crucial role. It is not difficult to have a younger-looking face at fifty or sixty, but the neck might show the aging effect very much at this age. Do not postpone your neck lift; remember that it is easier to prevent than to treat!

CHAPTER 9

Décolletage–One of the Signs of Photoaging

Does décolletage attract your attention? If not, skip this chapter. It will happen when you would like to open your décolletage but you feel uncomfortable with that. Rough texture, pigment spots, wrinkles, dry skin…we exposed this area to the sun and now pay the debt. It happens usually after the winter. You want to be exposed to the sun but feel "it is not for me anymore"—horrible thoughts in the brain. Do not worry; it is curable. The name of such a condition is solar elastosis. And I know how to handle it.

To Get Rid of Solar Skin Elastosis

In my practice, I see a lot of clients who just want to get rid of wrinkles in the areas of the upper lip, décolletage, neck, and hands. Most of my clients are age fifty and over, and their concerns are rough skin, deep creases, fine wrinkles, plaque-like thickening, yellowish skin color, and pigment spots especially in the areas of the neck, chest, hands, and around the mouth.

All of them represent the baby-boomer generation; they are people who have spent lots of time under the sun. Now they feel good, eat healthily, and are in good shape; their faces look as good as they want, and they are doing surgical and nonsurgical treatments, but...the neck and décolletage areas, areas around the mouth, and the hands are huge markers of their aging. The reason for this change is prolonged sun exposure with the developed condition called solar elastosis.

Clinical changes in sun-exposed skin, called photoaging, are characterized as changing the texture, color, and moisturizing level. The texture of the skin is rough. There are visible deep creases or many wrinkles. Some ladies see plaque-like thickening areas. The color of the skin changes to yellowish with irregular pigmentation. Some areas show red spots called *telangiectasia*. The skin feels and looks dry.

Changes in the texture include the following:

- Rough surface
- Deep creases
- Fine wrinkles
- Plaque-like thickening

The color changes are characterized by the following:

- A yellowish shadow
- Irregular pigmentation
- *Teleangiectasia*, caused by small broken capillaries

Skin dryness is a marker of photoaged skin's dehydration.

Medically speaking, all these changes are expressions of the thickness of the superficial skin layer with an increase in the number of pigment deposits. Looking under the microscope, we find tangled and thickened elastic fibers, a lot of deformed collagen, and not many cells that can produce new collagen, along with a very damaged capillary net around them.

All these clinical changes are reflected by such alterations of the skin as the following:

- The thickness of the superficial skin layer
- An increasing number of pigment cells
- An increasing number of tangled and thickened elastic fibers
- A lot of deformed collagen fibers
- A decreased amount of collagen
- Dehydration
- The lack of capillary blood flow

So many changes should be treated not in one but in a series of treatments. At least five or six treatments are required to see a good result.

The treatments that give this good result, especially in combination, are chemical peels, phototherapy, and laser resurfacing.

Chemical Peels

Since solar elastosis is skin damage in both levels of the skin—the dermis (collagen and elastin) and epidermis (dead cells and pigment cells)—the treatment should target both of them.

Superficial chemical peels work only on the level of the epidermis. Midlevel peels, such as retinol and TCA, have a maximum influence on the superficial layer of the dermis. Phenol peels, such as nonablative lasers, are able to stimulate changes on the level of the deep dermis. But one has to consider that the top skin layer has a lot of dead cells. This means that the way for a peel should be prepared. In order to allow the peel to go deeper into the superficial skin layer, mechanical removal of dead cells is recommended. Simply speaking, microdermabrasion prepares the way for deeper peel absorbing.

Phototherapy—Photofacial (IPL Technology)

IPL technology is able to change the skin color by interacting with pigment cells, but it can do nothing with the massive elastic conglomerates in the dermis. So, IPL therapy for décolletage skin elastosis is an additional tool to get the desired result, but it is far away from being the main one.

Laser Resurfacing

The fractional RF system is able to work on the level of the dermis, with damaged elastin and collagen fibers. Fractional RF also works on the level of superficial skin, stimulating the process of exfoliation and skin renewal.

Similar to laser action, a response of the tissues is achieved by using high-energy settings with short pulse durations. Thermal-zone injuries in the upper skin layer work to burn out the areas of dead cells and pigment deposits.

For skin rejuvenation, the same system but with a longer pulse duration is used. With a longer pulse, it is possible to deliver a sufficient dose of energy to the elastin- and collagen-degeneration areas. These areas will be destroyed by heat. Moreover, at the same time, the heat will stimulate cells producing fresh collagen and elastin to work intensively.

The result of such a smart combination will be a reduction of dark spots, even skin tone, skin tightening, and skin lifting.

It is a well-known fact that photoaged skin heals in a very bad way, first of all because of dehydration and the lack of capillary blood flow. Such serious skin stimulation as fractional RF will demand additional skin hydration afterward in order to reply to the damages created by the system. For this purpose, mesotherapy, needle or needle free, with hyaluronic acid is used. Hyaluronic acid, through raising the level of moisturizing, stimulates the recovery of tissues after the treatment.

The result is gradual. After the first treatment, skin looks much lighter and more even. After the second, clients feel the skin is smoother and see fewer wrinkles and creases. After the third session, it is an absolutely different skin. I would like to say it is time to buy necklaces!

CHAPTER 10

Injections, Threads, and PRP for Beauty

Neurotoxin and filler injections are now the most popular treatments that clients inquire about.

Clients ask the following questions when curious about the injection treatments:

- Are they safe? And how safe are they?
- How long do they last?
- Are they better than skin tightening?
- How much do they cost?

Before answering these questions about injections, it helps to clarify from the start. There are two *different* ways to work with the skin. The first is a total correction, and the second is a local correction.

Total correction is a skin-longevity treatment that is based on improving the skin condition. It means stimulation toward production of collagen and elastin, raising skin's hydration levels, and accelerating turnover of the epidermal cells. The examples of total correction are radiofrequency skin tightening, IPL photofacials, lasers, mesotherapy, and so on.

Neurotoxins, fillers, and threads are the usual tools for *local correction*. They diminish the depth of wrinkles and folds in the restricted areas. Specialists will tell you that threads and fillers will stimulate collagen production too. It is the truth. We expect collagen growth only in the particular area of injection.

Let's talk about the neurotoxin. It is a blocking agent that prevents intramuscular contraction. It has been represented on the market by many brand names; the most recognized are Botox, Dysport, Neuronox, Purtox, BTXA, and Xeomin. But the specialists call all of them neurotoxins. Neurologists began using neurotoxins in the middle of the last century. This fact demonstrates that the field of medicine has a proven track record of confirming the safety of the substances. Neurotoxins do not paralyze muscles, as many people think; they only interrupt the transmission of the impulse from one neuron to another for a period of time. Usually, this time frame is three to six months, and afterward, the muscle contracts, and no neurotoxin is found in the tissues.

In some situations, neurotoxins do not give the desired result. There are documented cases of clients showing complete or partial resistance to neurotoxins. According to statistics, on average, one in a hundred clients has such a resistance.

The effects of neurotoxin injections are felt in less active movements of some groups of muscles within one day to two weeks after the injections begin. This usually lasts three to six months. The length of effect depends on the following:

- The amount of substance in the injection
- The depth of the injection in the muscle, just under the skin, or inside of the skin
- The brand of the product

After the injections, you might be invited for a correction.

Correction should be done not more than two weeks after the injections. After two weeks, there should be no neurotoxin injections for three months. Three months after the first injection is called the *period of immunologic reactions*. If you have additional neurotoxin injections during this period of time, you might get a response of the resistance from your body. It is feasible to expect that neurotoxin injections will demonstrate results less than three months into the treatment, or you can expect the results to diminish when compared to the previous injections.

The most popular reasons for neurotoxin injections are the following:

- Horizontal forehead lines
- Vertical lines between the brows
- Crow's-feet
- Brow lowering
- Brow elevation
- Downward turning of the mouth
- Bunny lines on the side of the nose

- Vertical upper-lip lines
- Turkey necklines
- Horizontal necklines
- Excessive underarm, foot, or hand sweating

How to Determine If You Are a Good Candidate for These Injections?

You should be satisfied with the results if your muscles in these areas work actively and create wrinkles and you are younger than sixty-five years old. In this case, you are a good candidate. My advice is try it!

You begin to see the difference after a few days and often more so after two weeks. Please do not think after just ten days that it does not work. Be patient!

How Much Do You Need?

Trust the advice of a specialist. Tell her or him what your main goal is. How do you want your eyebrows to be lifted up? Do you want your forehead to have active movement or not? Draw the attention of the specialists to the areas around the eyes. In cases where your eyes are puffy, you often suffer from allergies. The bags under eyes appear and disappear seemingly without reason; emphasize these details to the injector.

Do not forget to mention the drugs that you take, even if you are not asked! Many medications—such as aminoglycosides, penicillamine quinine, and calcium channel blockers—decrease neuromuscular transmission and should be avoided in patients treated with neurotoxins.

To decrease the risk of bruising, avoid taking medications like ibuprofen (Advil, Motrin) or naproxen (Aleve).

Recommendations for after the injection include the following:

- Avoid sun exposure.
- Avoid taking ibuprofen, acetaminophen, and vitamin E.
- Avoid excessive physical activity for at least four hours.

Build Your Own Plan

- How do you want to look after the neurotoxin injections?
- Be informed about the price of the unit.
- Ask them to open the vial in front of you to ensure that the solution is fresh. After dissolving, it works for a limited period of time.
- Ask to be shown how many units will be injected in the insulin syringe.
- If it is more than fifty, you have to ask exactly how safe it is for you.
- When you book the appointment for the injections, inquire how much time you are going to spend with the injector. It should be at least thirty minutes.

Neurotoxins for the Body

Neurotoxins are a treatment option for the neck, décolletage, and scars.

For the neck treatments, the goal is to smooth out the cords, which appear as one of the signs of aging. Releasing a very specific muscle, called the platysma (partly attached to the bones and partly intertwined with the skin), is beneficial in reducing the appearance of cords. It is expected that fifty to a hundred units of neurotoxin will be injected to achieve the result. One or two weeks after the neurotoxin injection, you can expect to see cords diminished but not completely removed. This is because the neurotoxin works to relax the muscles and not intentionally to lift the skin. The fractional-radiofrequency system for the total correction (skin lifting) combined with the neurotoxin injection will give a much more impressive and needed result. I would recommend a treatment plan starting with the fractional RF and one to three treatments with an interval of one month between fractional RF sessions plus the neurotoxin for the décolletage lines and neck. Such a combination will make the appearance of these areas completely different and much younger looking.

Fillers

After clients began to inquire about filler injections, I realized that the biggest concern they have is a fear of looking unnatural. This section explains how the treatment works, what you can expect to see after the filler injections, and how to avoid an artificial look.

The goal for fillers is to make the skin lines smoother and wrinkles less prominent and to replace lost tissue volume. They may be used anywhere on the face—lips, nose, and around the mouth. For such purposes, different substances, namely hyaluronic acid, lactic acid, collagen, and even synthetic particles, are used. These substances might be injected into the skin, under the skin, or much deeper beneath the skin on top of the bones.

The objective for the injections is to reduce wrinkles, replace volume, hydrate the skin, or stimulate the process of collagen formation in the precise area of the injections.

To sum up, there are some differences that you should know about when you make a decision to be injected with fillers:

- The filler-injection substance
- The depth of the injection

- The number of syringe injections in each area for a natural look in each client
- What exactly is declared by a manufacturer

There are many different brands of dermal fillers on the market, and it is often difficult to know which fillers are the best for you and your concerns. The most popular dermal-filler brands are Restylane, Perlane, Juvéderm Ultra, Teosyal, Belotero, Radiesse, and Sculptra. All these dermal fillers work differently, and it is you and your injection provider's decision to determine the one that fits your individual needs.

All fillers are divided into two main groups: temporary and permanent. They are named after the substance base and the density of the substance.

Temporary Fillers

Most dermal fillers are considered to be safe products that are absorbed by the body over a period of six to nine months. They can be used to address various concerns, namely fine lines, wrinkles, folds, and volume loss. Temporary fillers are made from different kinds of man-made and synthetic materials, including hyaluronic acid, calcium hydroxylapatite, and collagen. The most common and popular are fillers with the hyaluronic acid.

Hyaluronic-Acid Fillers

Hyaluronic acid is a natural substance, present in every living organism. The body accepts products with hyaluronic acid as biocompatible, so they rarely cause any unwanted reactions.

The difference between HA fillers is not only the brand name; there are different thicknesses or viscosities. It is easy to realize that the thin skin layer under the eyes should be injected with a product of a low density, whereas if the objective is to increase the volume in the area of cheekbones, a product of high density should be used.

Specialists consider more factors that make these fillers different, but for the customer, this information is not really needed.

Some postinjection recommendations are to use ice to avoiding bruising and apply pressure immediately after the injections. Massaging the area after an injection will help reduce lumpiness. Some HA products will swell and feel firmer to palpation in the first week but blend in more naturally a bit later.

As previously described, RF technology is quite expeditious in correcting the prominent lumps, granulomas, and Tyndall effect—reflecting the filler by light that gives bluish hue.

Collagen Fillers

Collagen fillers were the first type of temporary filler used for cosmetic enhancement. These products are derived from bovine (cow) collagen.

We can only suppose that they trigger an allergic reaction in the body. That is why the manufacturers require an allergy test before treatment. However, newer products have the advantages of collagen injections without the need for pretesting. With the newest technology, porcini collagen is used. It has the properties of a natural collagen found in the skin. It does not require pretesting. The results of injection last for up to twelve months.

Calcium Hydroxylapatite

Calcium hydroxylapatite (CaHA) is a filler that stimulates collagen production. The filler consists of CaHA spheres suspended in an aqueous gel. This product has been used in dentistry for many years. In the field of aesthetic medicine, it is used in cheek, jaw, cranial, and chin areas. It is not recommended to apply the substance for treatment of lips or around the eyes.

This product improves severe folds and wrinkles. Calcium-hydroxylapatite filler is placed deeply under the skin. It is a longer-lasting but temporary dermal filler developed especially for facial sculpting. It is also quite popular for injections in deep mouth lines and nose reshaping. But it's never used for lip treatments.

Poly-L-Lactic Acid as a Collagen Stimulator

This product is used to restore volume in faces that have developed lipoatrophy from aging or using HIV medications. It is also a product for improving deep folds and lines. After injections of this substance, it is advised to massage the injected areas for five minutes five times a day for five days in order to avoid occlusion or compression of the tissues.

The most well-known PLLA collagen stimulator works to encourage formation of own collagen. In addition, it similarly influences the dermal fillers. This product not only adds volume, like traditional fillers, but also improves skin texture and tone by stimulating new collagen growth in the areas of injections. The effects of PLLA filler can last for up to two years and occur gradually over several months, making the results more subtle. The fact that the result is not immediately noticeable makes this product enticing for women, who wish to avoid looking like they had something *done*.

Permanent Fillers

Polymethyl-Methacrylate (PMMA)

These are not as widely used as temporary fillers. Because of the semipermanence of this product, it should be injected only for the improvement of the nasolabial folds, cheeks or midface, and marionette lines.

The synthetic substance polymethylmethacrylate is made from a mixture of tiny plastic (methylmethacrylate) microspheres suspended in collagen gel.

This substance is injected very deep underneath the skin. Over time, these very small plastic beads become encapsulated in collagen tissues. The collagen holds the plastic beads in place and does not allow them to move.

The effect can last from months to years before the collagen disperses. If you are thinking of having a permanent filler, make sure you go to someone who is very experienced with using the product. As you might realize, there is no way to restore the tissue to a previous state, and any overinjected area will be visible for many years.

Before you are injected with the permanent fillers, I advise you to try out treatments with temporary products, ensuring that you are happy with the result.

How Much Do I Need?

This is really a difficult question. The amount and density of a substance are discussed with a specialist during your consultation. Everyone is concerned about being overinjected. If you are really concerned about the way you will look after the injections, begin a treatment with one syringe injection only. You will never look fake with that amount.

In many cases, clients notice the results immediately and return to the clinic two weeks after the injections just for a checkup. You could also add as many syringes to your desired area as you want. In your next visit, the specialist will correct the asymmetry if it happened after the previous injection or if it was not completely corrected with the first injection.

Please remember that in most cases, the first result of the filler injection will be visible immediately, but further results appear in a couple of weeks and the final result one month after the first filler injection. Filler injections are a method of local correction and the fastest way to diminish the appearance of wrinkles and folds and replace volume to look much younger.

Mesotherapy

Mesotherapy treatment is the delivery of minerals, proteins, and vitamins to the middle layer of the skin, the dermis. There are two methods of such a delivery—with needles or without needles. Here we will talk about delivery using needles.

Mesotherapy treatment is a cosmetic solution for such body concerns as cellulite, excess weight, and body contouring. Distinct results can be expected only by combining it with lymphatic massage, ultrasound, or radiofrequency. For the face and neck areas, mesotherapy plays the role of one more tool for tissue stimulation.

Mesotherapy works through the process of wound healing and the delivery of active substances into the skin. Technically, mesotherapy is the small wounds made with needles. It might be a single needle attached to the syringe with the mesotherapeutic solution or a simple device with many needles, called a derma pen. The basic principle of both is the delivery of the products into the skin. It is not true that mesotherapy does not create pain. Any puncture by a needle creates pain, but every individual has a different bearable pain level.

PRP

What Is PRP?

Platelet-rich plasma (PRP) is a high concentration of human platelets in a small volume of plasma. The PRP effect is based on the fundamental protein growth factors. Protein growth factor is actively secreted by platelets to initiate all wound-healing processes. The biologically active signal peptides released from the platelet fraction initiate a normal wound-healing process that triggers new vessel formation and collagen stimulation.

Is PRP Treatment Safe?

The therapy based on enriched plasma injections was used very successfully in the second part of the twentieth century. The reason behind its success was the stimulation of the body's immune system to battle with acne. Studies showed an improvement in the healing of soft tissues after the plasma injections reached these areas. Moreover, as PRP is created from a patient's own blood, it is considered a relatively low-risk and natural treatment with the potential to improve or speed up the healing process.

How Is It Done?

The blood is taken from a vein. Then it is put into a vial and centrifuged. This separates the red and white blood cells and platelets. Platelets, which are part of the blood, are the PRP substance injected under the skin of the face or scalp.

After the surgery, laser treatment, or fractional-radiofrequency treatment, it is common to just spread the plasma over the damaged skin.

The result is expected three weeks after the treatment. An immediate result is only possible with using PRP and filler injections in one treatment.

Threading

Threading is one of the more popular antiaging techniques. Threading deals with three major objectives:

1. Skin lifting—soft-tissue lifting
2. Skin framing—skin fixation at a precise position or location
3. Biological stimulation of the skin cells with the goal of collagen and elastin production

The effect of threading includes skin lifting and support. This treatment can be used on the face, neck, décolletage, and on the various areas of the body.

How Do Threads Work?

Threads are alien to skin tissue. Their presence in the skin initiates a process of the body's response to a foreign body. This response means minimal inflammatory process with the result of collagen and elastin production and formation of the connective bands.

Modern threads are completely synthetic products made from the following:

- Polylactic acid
- Caprolacton
- Polydioxanon
- Polyglyconids and their polymers

The effect of treatment depends on how soon the thread will resolve in a body. If the thread is resolving very rapidly, the tissues are not able to respond with the effect of the formation of connective support.

The type of biodegradation depends on the thickness of a thread, the number of threads, the type of threads, the point of insertion, and the individual metabolic processes of the body.

The manufacturers of different threads promise different long-lasting effects. Practice shows that the response of the tissue and the effect are individual.

In order to get better and longer-lasting results, skin should be prepared for such an invasive technology. It is common sense that skin after forty should be stimulated to produce new collagen and elastin before the threading. It is also recommended to have good moisturizing of skin on deep and superficial levels to respond properly to the treatment. RF skin tightening and mesotherapy, especially with injections of peptides, are the fastest way to prepare the tissue for thread lifting.

There are lots of discussions on the market in the last two years about the results versus complications of threads.

CHAPTER 11

An Easy Way to Get Rid of Cellulite

Eighty percent of all clients who come for body treatments mention cellulite as their main concern.

"Cellulite is not a necessary part of women's bodies. It forms as a result of excess acids and toxins, which sometimes the body is not able to remove. The body safely deals with this toxic backup and tries to neutralize these metabolic products by surrounding them with mucus and then storing them as far as possible from your precious organs and glands, just under the skin. These pockets of fat and mucus are clearly visible on thighs, arms, and buttocks as the fatty, puckery deposits women's hate" (Wiseman, 2012).

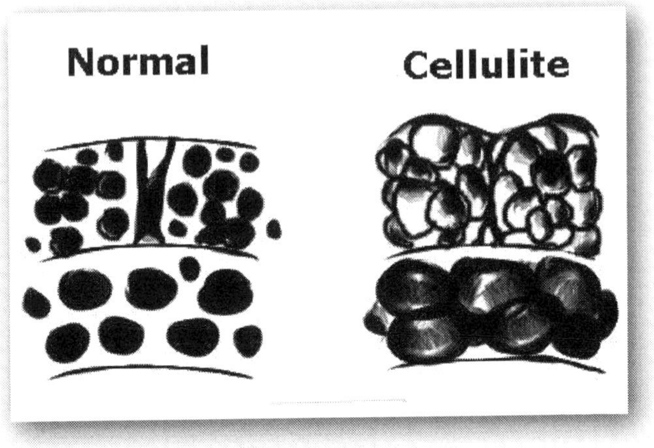

What Is Cellulite?

Cellulite is a very common aesthetic condition in women in whom the skin acquires an orange-peel or mattress appearance. Cellulite is the result of a number of metabolic changes:

- Insufficient capillary function and diminishing microcirculation, meaning that the process of the delivery of nutrients and oxygen to the skin suffers
- An impaired venous-lymphatic system (venous lymphatic edema), meaning that body does not remove waste products and fluids properly; the result of such

an impaired function is edema or tissue swelling
- Growing fat cells, called adipocytes, and increasing water in the fat tissues (lipoedema)
- Inflammation and fibrosis in connective tissues and fat tissues—being under the pressure of liquid and waste products and not sufficiently supplied with oxygen and nutrients, tissues ask the body for help through the process of inflammation
- Sagging body skin

Why Do Women Have Cellulite?

Fat cells grow in size not only because of fat deposits but also because of the increase in the remaining liquid in the fat cells. The lymphatic system and circulatory system are not able to get rid of the body's excess fluids and metabolic products in the way that they should. Oversized fat cells suppress microcirculation. The result is as follows: deficient blood flow, liquid remaining in the tissues with metabolic products (toxins for the body), oversized fat cells, and tissue-fibrotic changes (tough bumps).

Who Is Predisposed to Have Cellulite?

There are some groups of conditions and factors that demonstrate a predisposition to cellulite:

- Family history—hereditary endocrine-metabolic syndromes and common nutritional deficiencies
- Body structure—postural and spinal-column alterations, as these problems are associated with inadequate footwear
- Hormone-dependent conditions—patients suffering from hormone dysfunction, patients taking estroprogestagens, such as in birth-control pills and food preservatives, stimulating interstitial liquid retention
- Food—patients consuming estrogen or hormone-supplemented food and excesses of sugar and fat
- Somatic disorders—intestinal flora disorders

- Behavior—external compression, such as tight clothing, inhibiting the lymphatic and microcirculatory systems by creating metabolic hypoxia; sedentary lifestyle; poor diet; obesity or having constipation; and smoking, which slows down microcirculation in the cutaneous arterioles and creates tissues hypoxia

To determine if the person is predisposed to having cellulite or enhanced cellulite appearance with age, it is recommended to consider the following:

- The age of onset of cellulite
- Family history (it is very common that women have cellulite if their mother does)
- Prior occurrence of trauma or surgery (e.g., disc removal)
- Liposuction in the affected area
- Presence of chronic vascular or associated hormonal diseases

- Occasional or regular use of medications, including hormonal treatments
- A sedentary lifestyle, certain food habits, psychosomatic factors, smoking

Understand the Stage of Cellulite

In front of the mirror, using fingers, try to squeeze the skin. At the same time, measure the skin temperature with the palms.

Stage 1

1. Does squeezed skin resemble an orange peel?
2. Do some body areas appear to have a pale color?

Stage 2

1. Is squeezing or applying pressure on the skin painful?
2. Are prominences and hollows visible without squeezing?

Stage 3

1. Are some nodes on the surface of the skin visible?
2. Is touching them painful?
3. Does the skin have a bluish color?
4. Is the skin cold upon touching?
5. Does it show tissue edema or tissue fibrosis?

Such tests help us to realize what stage the cellulite is in.

To understand cellulite better, practitioners should ask what plays the most significant role in a particular case of cellulite. Is this factor fibrotic tissue, tissue swelling, an increase in the size of fat cells, bad lymphatic drainage, or the insufficient supply of tissues with oxygen and nutrients because of impaired circulation?

Understanding the process of cellulite appearance and triggering factors for the cellulite in each particular case helps to get results for cellulite treatment reasonably fast and guarantees a client's satisfaction.

Cellulite treatment should have the following objectives:

- Restoring local microcirculation by improving the oxygen and nutrition supplies of the tissues
- Increasing venolymphatic drainage and removing accumulated fluids and toxins
- Increasing lipolytic activity (physiological lipolysis) and metabolic exchanges
- Decreasing interstitial edema or swelling
- Diminishing fibrosis
- Stimulating collagen growth activity

According to Jean-Marc Chardonneau's classification, which I see as the most practically useful, there are following types of cellulite:

1. Edema cellulite
2. Muscle-aponeurotic cellulite
3. Adiposa cellulite
4. Fibrotic cellulite
5. Atonic cellulite

1. Edema Cellulite

This is the orange-peel skin. Clients see holes on the skin after touching it. The legs feel heavy. Typically, people who have this kind of cellulite mention they also have intestinal disturbances, such as disbakteriosis or irritable bowel syndrome (IBS).

The reasons for this type of cellulite are hormonal changes, which result in gluten and lactose deficiencies. Incorrect food chewing is one of the reasons mentioned by the specialists.

The treatment plan is based on a minimum of fifteen treatments using vacuum mechanical massage as well as probiotics and food-behavior changes.

In addition, the following are recommended:

- A decrease in consumption of meat and dairy products and avoiding high-protein diets
- No late-evening meals
- Proper chewing patterns—hard food should be chewed thoroughly before it is mixed with saliva completely and swallowed

The treatment plan will focus on improving blood and lymphatic circulation, for example, using vacuum mechanical or vacuum-roller massage.

2. Muscle-Aponeurotic Cellulite

It is quite common for women who are active and involved in sports to have this type of cellulite. Impaired lymphatic drainage, in this case, is the result of growing muscles. Simply speaking, muscles press the lymphatic vessels. The result is the liquid remaining inside the tissues, tissue swelling, and cellulite.

The treatment plan includes lymphatic-drainage massage (it is better when the massage is done in conjunction with a system). This is *the only solution* for this type of cellulite.

3. Adiposa Cellulite (Soft Cellulite)

Women with excessive weight commonly have this type of cellulite. It is a result of a "sluggish" lymphatic system due to hypodynamic behavior and excessive food consumption.

The treatment plan includes the following:

- Decreasing the amount of food and calories
- Increasing physical activity, including walking or going to the gym
- Deep-tissue massage—mechanical systems compared with manual systems are more successful because of the depth of penetration
- Injections or needle-free delivery into the skin the substances forcing lipolysis or fat removal

4. Fibrotic Cellulite

Before fibrosis appears, tissues will go through the long-lasting process of edema. Fibrotic cellulite is the last stage of the cellulites, as mentioned before. Sometimes, fibrotic cellulite is the consequence of liposuction. Fibrotic cellulite shows up as bumps on the skin. This cellulite is more localized when compared to others and often painful.

For the treatment plan, the main goal is fibrotic-tissue destruction. For this purpose, vacuum mechanical massage for the start of the program is used. After a few sessions, treatment with radiofrequency technology is recommended. A combination of vacuum mechanical massage with RF treatment in one procedure is the best solution for handling fibrotic cellulite.

Needle-free mesotherapy works as a booster for this type of cellulite, delivering lipolytics, peptides, and hyaluronic acid into the tissues. Lipolytics work as fat resolvers. Peptides work as collagen boosters. Hyaluronic acid is a strong moisturizer, helping all these processes work in a better way.

From the perspective of food behavior, to be successful in improving the fibrotic cellulite, it is highly recommended to decrease consumption of simple carbohydrates.

5. Atonic Cellulite

"This type of cellulite affects slender women with underdeveloped muscular systems. It also attacks aging ladies with an attic skin. From a physiology perspective, there is no cellulite. Uneven skin is a result of bumpy hypodermis with lobed fat skin layer under the thin, sagging, nonelastic skin."[2]

This type of cellulite is the most difficult one to treat. To correct this condition, it is necessary to improve skin quality and microcirculation. The use of radiofrequency technology provides the best result, increasing the thickness of the skin.

However, the RF effect lasts for a certain time period; hence, a maintenance program is strongly recommended. The maintenance treatments can also be replaced with vacuum mechanical massage technologies scheduled on a frequent basis.

Treatments should be provided on a regular basis because the main reason for skin atony is insufficient deep-tissue circulation and often lack of skin hydration. As skin is predisposed to these conditions, external stimulation should be performed.

2 Jean-Marc Chardonneau (2013).

Summary: How to Treat Cellulite

There are strategies available for the successful treatment of cellulite. Because the main concern with the appearance of cellulite is a problem with microcirculation, the step 1 is improvement of microcirculation. Activation of microcirculation helps to activate fast drainage and lipolytic processes, using the natural body systems of regulation.

It is a well-known fact that the best and quickest way to stimulate microcirculation and lymphatic drainage is a vacuum mechanical massage. Hand massage is also good, but it isn't comparable with the massage performed with modern systems. Modern machines are developed especially for stimulation of deep drainage and microcirculation. Massages with systems not only improve the flow of lymph with waste products but also increase the vein outflow from the lower extremities and increase cellular respiration.

Step 2 is stimulation of lipolysis. Basically, lipolysis means that the fat cells should be decreased in size. It is possible to shrink fat cells with the use of various technologies, such as radiofrequency, ultrasound, cryolypolysis, and lymphatic massage.

Step 3 is collagen formation. Collagen rebuilds structures called septa inside the fat skin layer and shrinks the fibrosis area. Radiofrequency is the treatment of choice for this purpose.

Step 4 is the most important. All these steps result in the positive outcome the clients seek but only if they are combined with lymphatic-drainage massage. Preferably, this massage is done with systems, not hands.

Don't believe the marketing ads that offer you fast and permanent results for cellulite treatment. I would like to make it very clear that we constantly struggle with cellulite. We celebrate the victory only for a period of time. Skin physiology and the function of the lymphatic system make it impossible to have permanent results. Also, please don't forget that cellulite is not only an aesthetic condition but also a sign of body toxicity and bad microcirculation.

CHAPTER 12

Getting Rid of Saggy Arm Skin

For women, arms are especially visible when it is necessary to wear cocktail dresses or summer clothes without sleeves. Why does the skin in the arm area show age faster compared with that of other body parts? It happens because the inner sides of the arms have thinner skin and are less hydrated. These two factors speed up the aging process. Moreover, the body shape significantly depends on the muscle frame, which is weak in this area. The muscle frame loses strength every ten years; it is a law.

Thus, aging in the arms can be explained by changes in the depth of skin, fat, and muscles. Skin loses its elasticity and stretches out. It appears as skin sagginess, skin folds, and stretch marks. Repositioning of the fat with concentration in some areas builds folds under the arms. Lymphatic-flow insufficiency and edema are reasons for the cellulite or "bumpy arms." Atony and dystrophy of muscles underline the arms' aging.

People are looking for help with arms after forty. The earlier the better does not work for the arms. Sometimes results at the age of sixty are more impressive compared with those at forty. The result of treatments depends on the reasons for aging in this area.

When the main reason is clarified, an individual program should be built. The program usually consists of two parts. First, efforts are implemented on the level of soft tissues like skin and fat. The second goal is working on other levels that potentiate the effect and prevent the future aging changes.

Methods of Correction

Even ten years ago, the one way to correct aging in the area of the upper arms was brachioplasty.

Brachioplasty is a plastic-surgery method in which the excessive amount of skin is removed. Modern aesthetic medicine offers many therapeutic ways to correct these changes. The majority of clients prefer therapy to plastic surgery just because of the decreased risks and downtime.

Methods of upper-arm aging correction might be divided into three different groups based on the particular goals:

1. Arms skin tightening
2. Fat removal
3. Changing the muscle frame

1. Arms skin tightening

Skin loses elasticity because of storage of damaged collagen and the slowing down of new collagen synthesis. These changes are shown as sagging skin in the inner-arm area. Lower levels of hydration compared with other body parts are a predisposing factor that make arm conditions worse.

Total and local corrections should be considered when the goal is to improve skin elasticity in the underarm area.

The method of choice from the perspective of total correction is RF skin tightening, which destroys damaged collagen and stimulates new collagen synthesis. It is recommended to have six sessions with one to two weeks in between them. To reinforce the result of skin tightening, deep skin hydration with mesotherapy should be used. Delivery of peptides and hyaluronic acid reinforces the processes of restoring skin elasticity. Peptides work as collagen boosters, and hyalyronic acid is a direct skin moisturizer. There are two kinds of mesotherapy—with needles and needle free—that give very comparable results.

Threading for the vector displacement of tissues is the preferable technology for local correction. There are two types of threads that are used for this area. The first one is polydioxanone threads, which are inserted into the skin at the depth between skin and under-skin fat layers, building the frame. The threads are replaced by connective-tissue bands that raise skin thickness.

Polydioxanone threads are dissolved by the body completely within six to eight months.

Implantation of the threads of polylactic acid and polycaprolactone, which are known as remodeling threads, has a more irritating and stimulating influence on the tissues compared with that of polydioxanone threads. The result of such insertion is a frame of collagen tissues with a higher density. Polylactic acid and polycaprolactone threads are placed in the level of under-skin fat. They are fixed with the notches, spikes, and cones that these types of threads usually have. The threads are completely biodegradable within a year.

Clients older than seventy are not the best candidates for the thread technologies, and they get more benefits when their treatment plan includes not only radiofrequency (RF) and mesotherapy but also fractional RF as an additional tool for skin tightening.

2. Fat removal

Working with the fat skin layer has only one goal: decreasing the fat layer through a process called lipolysis and lymphatic drainage. It is possible to divide the methods for therapeutic lipolysis into three different groups:

1. Systems or technologies that work for lypolysis
2. Injections that work as lypolytics
3. Systems that stimulate lymphatic drainage

Technologies That Work for Fat Cells

There are some different technologies that work on the level of fat cells, but a tremendous result is not expected after one session with any system.

The most popular of them are RF and ultrasound cavitation.

RF technology is based on raising the temperature up to 43°C in the depth of the fat layer and maintaining the temperature for ten minutes, which starts the process of lypolysis. The treatment protocol demands six treatments to shrink the fat layer. Only some RF technologies work on the lymphatic drainage directly. These are systems that combine RF and vacuuming.

Ultrasound cavitation or acoustic cavitation is the method of influencing fat cells. It is recommended to have six to ten treatments for the upper-arm area.

Massage with Systems for Fat Removal

There are not many such systems on the market. From the perspective of having long-lasting results, they are considered as the treatments of choice. It is recommended to have a minimum of fifteen treatments, which have the goal of starting a lypolytic process, increasing the temperature in the precise area as well as stimulating lymphatic drainage.

Injections

Desoxycholat is the main substance that aesthetic medicine uses in order to stimulate lypolysis. Many injections in the depth of fat cells with special needles are provided. The number of treatments is two or more with an interval of three weeks. Bruising is expected.

Systems That Stimulate Lymphatic Drainage

There are several of them on the market. Some of them use rollers and some cups. The most updated systems combine vacuuming, cups, and rollers. Vacuums work for lymphatic drainage, removing excessive water and products of the metabolism. Such a body detox works as a trigger for normalizing the processes of fat storage and fat resolving and reasonably provides the long-lasting result of fat removal. Modern cups (which are as different from the old as a smartphone is from just a phone) and rollers help lymph to flow, normalizing metabolism.

3. Working with Muscles

Aesthetic medicine offers a program of electrical myostimulation, but specialists consider this way of working with muscles as not primary but subsidiary. Physical activity, as proved, is the best way for restoring muscle structure.

A Comprehensive Approach for the Correction of the Upper-Arm Area

To find the best, fastest, and longest-lasting way of correcting the upper-arm area, the depth of changes (skin, fat, and muscles) should be considered. Distinguishing the main reason for changes (skin, fat, or lymphatic stack) helps to establish the right goal for treatment. Successful treatment will be shown as tightened skin under the arms with less fat. It is a time to wear dresses without sleeves!

CHAPTER 13

A Desirable Result—A Flat Stomach

The stomach is the point of concern for most of women after forty. Periods of hormonal changes, pregnancies, and gain-loss weight periods reflect changes. The aging process changes the area of the stomach too; in addition to sagging skin, clients see fat deposits, called fat traps, in the abdominal area. Stretch marks on the stomach, decreases in skin density and elasticity, and fat deposits are reasons for clients' concern.

This area is the most difficult in getting satisfying results for clients. According to statistics, about 50 percent of clients have unrealistic expectations. They want flat stomachs without any folds, like the movie stars on the glossy magazine covers. To satisfy the clients, media and marketing offer visible and excellent results after a single treatment. But medically speaking, only surgery can offer such fast results. In other cases, combinations of techniques and technologies, based on treatments numbering six or more, can change the abdominal area's appearance.

There are two directions for the treatment plan. The first is fat elimination from the area. Different technologies, such as radiofrequency technology, ultrasound, and electrolypolysis, might work for such a goal. None of them, unfortunately, can give a really visible result after one treatment. The client should consider a series of treatments for two months or more.

The second is sagging-skin removal. Not only technologies but also threads and injections are used for this purpose. The name "skin tightening" by itself means that technologies called RF replace sagging skin with firmer skin. Polydioxanon threads after the RF series work well by continuously stimulating the collagen-formation process. Manufacturers usually recommend twenty to thirty threads for the abdominal area, which biologically degrade in a period of time from 120 to 240 days. During the period of this biological degradation, threads stimulate the new collagen growth process and raise skin elasticity. One more technical tool that is used with the goal of destroying collagen cross-links and boosting the collagen-formation process is needle or needle-free mesotherapy with insertion into the middle skin layer's peptides or DMAE (dimethylaminoethanol).

The real result is an absolutely different look in clothes and bikinis. It creates a body shape that you like in the mirror.

CHAPTER 14

Perfect Thighs

Manual massages for body corrections are still popular. They work well but not for all body areas. Some areas are too deep to respond to manual massage techniques. They definitely demand machines included in the treatment plans. One such part of the body that requires deep touching into the tissues is the thigh.

The thigh area is divided by specialists into specific zones:

- Knee
- Upper one-third of the outer thighs
- Upper part of the inner thighs
- Buttock area

Most clients who consider the thigh area as the main concern complain about cellulite or extremely saggy skin.

Aesthetic-medicine specialists see this problem as a wider one and consider it to involve cellulite, swelling, local fat deposits, sagging skin, and low muscle tone.

Individual treatment protocols should be built considering all the facts mentioned here.

Cellulite

Cellulite is such a common condition for clients that one of the chapters of this book is devoted to it.

Swelling

Touching the skin is painful for such clients. Tissues are so tight that it is impossible to fold them. One of the difficulties for manual therapists is the problem of reaching the depth of the interstitial space where a lot of fluid is deposited. Technologies reach such a depth easily with vacuuming and new forms of cups. Swelling is solved much more quickly with such technologies.

Fat Traps

After some treatments, clients mention looser jeans or smaller sizes of the clothes. It happens when tissue swelling is gone and body size is decreased. Very often, clients start to feel and see some soft bumps under the skin at this time. Bumps appear when the swelling is gone and fat pockets become visible. It is a time to work on the level of the fat. Working with fat is somewhat painful.

Skin

When edema is gone and the fat amount is decreased, clients pay attention to excessive skin. They pay attention mostly in the inner thigh and abdominal areas. It is very reasonable to include RF technology in addition to vacuum-system massage. Vacuum roller or vacuum mechanical massage prepares thighs for the RF treatment, improving blood circulation; blood is a conductive tissue for RF technology. The result of RF skin tightening followed by vacuum massage will be seen by clients even after the first treatment.

Muscles

Improving the muscle tone is the goal of physical activity.

Thighs really can look much thinner and younger. It is not difficult to change the shape of thighs using a combination of technologies. It just demands time. And you will enjoy your beauty wearing shorts and skirts.

CHAPTER 15

How to Get Rid of Back Folds and Buffalo Hump

Fat on the Back (Back Folds, Buffalo Hump)

To remove fat from the back with diet or physical activity is rarely possible. Clinical experience and research show that there are many body changes that facilitate the back fat deposits. To remove fat deposits in the areas of love handles, back folds, and shoulders, a comprehensive treatment approach should be used.

Back Folds

One of the issues of imperfection in the area of the back is back folds. Back folds consist of skin with fat under it. It has been medically proven that back folds are the consequence of changes in the thoracic spine. Wearing very tight (incommodious) bras and gravity make the situation worse.

All of the above creates stacks in the lymph flow and makes microcirculation in the area worse.

Lymphatic stasis, impaired microcirculation, and atony of muscles in the area are tissue changes that should be fixed in order to get rid of back folds.

Because of the different mechanisms causing folds' appearance, a combination of different technologies will be necessary to get results.

The targets for the back-folds treatment will be the lymphatic system, the vascular system, fat cells, skin, and muscles.

Treatment protocols should be started with technologies that improve lymphatic drainage and microcirculation. A combination of rollers and vacuum aspiration as a part of mechanical massage is the treatment of choice of specialists. To reinforce the fat-removal process, it is recommended to use technologies. Radiofrequency technology, ultrasound, and electrolypolysis can be performed to stimulate the process of lipolysis in the particular areas.

Mesotherapy might be considered as a booster to any of these technologies for the fat-removal process, but definitely not instead of them. Skin-tightening treatments are a good choice for the back-folds areas without excessive fat deposits. Muscle strength is under the responsibility of a personal trainer.

The treatment plan consists of fifteen to thirty treatments. Treatments should be started with one or two treatments per week, intensifying the program with two or three treatments per week. Each treatment might include one or two or a maximum of three ways to influence the tissues (different technologies and injections).

Buffalo Hump

Fat deposits in the area of the seventh cervical vertebra, called buffalo hump, is typical for women and for men as well. The difference is in the causes that create such a concern. These are some of the most significant triggers for buffalo hump:

1. Being overweight—increasing fat deposits in the upper part of the body (the abdominal type).
2. Premenopausal and menopausal hormonal changes are the reasons for the fat deposits in the upper part of the body (arms, shoulders, seventh cervical vertebra). Women who are genetically predisposed to being overweight will see the first fat deposits exactly in these areas.
3. Posture.
4. Thyroid gland–function changes—each organ has its projection in the vertebrae, and it is a well-known fact. The seventh cervical vertebra is the area of the projection of the thyroid gland. Any changes in this area might be markers for thyroid-gland dysfunction.

The main goal to work with for the seventh cervical vertebra is a local lipolysis. Because of the location, treatments with some systems are prohibited, and RF technology is chosen as the safest and most effective for this area. RF treatment increases the metabolic processes inside of fat cells and improves the processing of the released fatty acids through the cells' membranes. All these are called nonstraight lipolytic processes. RF energy does not hit the fat cells directly. RF raises the temperature in the septa that surround fat cells. It explains why the process of the fat cells' destruction is not impetuous and demands the concentration of a hit in the area of treatment. According to the treatment protocol, it is recommended to focus on an area of ten to fifteen square centimeters for ten to fifteen minutes. After the fat dissolves, the products of metabolism flow away with the lymph fluid. But they might be trapped by the areas not far from the seventh vertebra. According to the article of the St. Petersburg Institute of Beauty, a low fat diet should be chosen two days before the treatment, on the day of the treatment, and two days after in order to avoid recaptivation of free fatty acids by fat cells in the surrounding area. The recommended number of treatments is six to ten, once per week.

Usually after the second or third treatment with RF technology, the amount of the local fat decreases. Then it becomes reasonable to bring in the lipolytic cocktails using needle or needle-free mesotherapy. The number of lipolytic sessions is two or three, combined with a series of RF treatments.

In closing, the age of your skin is not the same as your passport age. It is the ability of the skin to resist certain factors that force us to look older. That would include sun, some foods, as well as natural aging. Wrinkles, pigment spots, rosacea, and cellulite are all a response to these factors. But not all skin responds equally. Skin with low resistance levels responds faster and shows much more signs of aging. On the other hand, skin with high resistance levels rebel against such factors and remains youthful. To keep yourself younger looking, your skin should be stimulated and trained. Trained skin has high immunity, and it is prepared to reply to harmful factors and resist them. Start working on it now to look younger longer!

BIBLIOGRAPHY

Adebamowo, C.A., D. Spiegelman, C. S. Berekey, F. W. Danby, H. H. Rockett, G. A. Colditz, W. C. Willett, and M. D. Holmes. 2006. "Milk Consumption and Acne in Adolescent Girls." *Dermatology Online Journal* 12 (4): 1.

Adebamowo, C. A., D. Spiegelman, C. S. Berkey, F. W. Danby, H. H. Rockett, G. A. Colditz, W. C. Willett, and M. D. Holmes. 2008. "Milk Consumption and Acne in Teenaged Boys." *Journal of the American Academy of Dermatology* 58 (5): 787–93.

Alexiades-Armenakas, M., D. Rosenberg, B. Renton, J. Dover, and K. Arndt. 2010. "Blinded, Randomized, Quantitative Grading Comparison of Minimally Invasive, Fractional Radiofrequency and Surgical Face-lift to Treat Skin Laxity." *Arch Dermatology*. www.archdermatology.com.

Al-Niaimi, F. 2014. "Revisiting Acne Vulgaris." *PRIME* 4:30–36.

Archer, C. B., S. N. Cohen, and S. E. Baron. 2012. "British Association of Dermatologists and Royal College of General Practitioners. Guidance on the Diagnosis and Clinical Management of Acne." *Clinical and Experimental Dermatology* 37 (Suppl 1): 1–6.

Belaya, N., and A. Lyutkevich. 1/2015. *Kompleksnaya korrektsiya lokalnych zhirovyh otlozheniy v oblasti spiny*. Gaggenau, Germany: Kosmetik International.

Belenkaya, I., M. Elman, U. B. Iosef, S. D. Brown, and M. Vashkevich. 1/2012. *Istoriya primeneniya RF-energii v esteticheskoy medicine*. Les Nouvelles Esthetiques Ukraine.

Belenkaya, I., M. Elman, U. B. Iosef, S. D. Brown, M. Vashkevich, and K. Levit. 4/2011: 705-721. "Radiochastotnaya terapiya v esteticheskoy medicine. Obsor." *Journal of Plastic Surgery and Cosmetology*

Belenkaya, I., M. Vashkevich, and K. Levit. 6/2011. *RF-apparaty: obosnovanie vybora*. Les Nouvelles Esthetiques.

Belenkaya, I., M. Elman, U. B. Iosef, S. D. Brown, M. Vashkevich, and K. Levit. 1/2012. "Radioterapiya I ee primenenie v esteticheskoy medicine." *Eksperimentalnaya & Klinicheskaya Dermatokosmetologiya*.p 6-16

Chardonneau, J. M. 3/2013. *Tipologiya cellulita: teooriya I praktika*. Les Nouvelles Esthetiques.

Clatici, V. G. 2014. "Acne in Adult Women: More Common and More Frustrating." *PRIME: International Journal of Aesthetic and Anti-ageing Medicine*. www.prime-journal.com.

Crowe, F. L., T. J. Key, N. E. Allen, and Others. 2009. "The Association between Diet and

Serum Concentrations of IGF-I, IGFBP-1, IGFBP-2, and IGFBP-3 in the European Prospective Investigation into Cancer and Nutrition." *Cancer Epidemiology, Biomarkers & Prevention* 18:1333–40.

Dahl, M.V. 2011. "Understanding and Addressing the Pathophysiology of Inflammation in Rosacea." *Medscape Nurses.* www.medscape.org.

Danby, F. W. 2005. "Acne and Milk, the Diet Myth, and Beyond." *Journal of the American Academy of Dermatology* 52 (2): 360–2.

Degitz, K., M. Placzek, C. Borelli, and G. Plewig. 2007. "Pathophysiology of Acne." *Journal der Deutschen Dermatologischen Gesellschaft* 5 (4): 316–23.

Del Rosso, J. Q., DO. 3/2010. "Rosacea—Myths and Realities: An Expert Interview with James Q. Del Rosso, DO." *Medscape Nurses.* www.medscape.org.

Duhanin, A. 1/2014. *Topicheskie preparaty dlya lecheniya akne: sostavnye chasti effektivnosti.* Gaggenau, Germany: Kosmetik International.

Ernandes, E. I., and A. A. Margolina. 2005. *Novaya kosmetologiya.* Moscow Kosmetika & Medicina.

Fedyakova, E. 2/2015. *Plazmoterapiya: endogennyj podhod k regeneratsii kozhi.* Gaggenau, Germany: Kosmetik International.

Hoppe, C., A. Vaag, V. Barkholt, and K. F. Michaelsen. 2005. "High Intakes of Milk, but not Meat, Increase s-insulin and Insulin Resistance in 8-year- Old Boys." *European Journal of Clinical Nutrition* 59 (3): 393–8.

Hoyt, G., M. S. Hickey, and L. Cordain. 2005. "Dissociation of the Glycaemic and Insulinaemic Responses to Whole and Skimmed Milk." *British Journal of Nutrition* 93 (2): 175–7.

Ignateva, A., I. Charyshneva, and N. Kalashnikova. 1/2015. *Korrekciya plech: vozmozhnosti terapevticheskoy kosmetologii.* Gaggenau, Germany: Kosmetik International.

Jesitus, J. 2014. "Filler Lift a Result of More than G-Prime." *The Dermatology Times*, April 1, 2014. http://dermatologytimes.modernmedicine.com/dermatology-times/news/filler-lift-result-more-g-prime.

Katsambas, A., and C. Dessinioti. 2014. "Melasma: The Most Common Pigmentary Disorder." *PRIME: International Journal of Aesthetic and Anti-ageing Medicine*. www.prime-journal.com.

Kligman, A. M. 1974. "An Overview of Acne." *Journal of Investigative Dermatology* 62:268–87.

Kolgunenko, I. I. 1974. "Osnovy geronto-kosmetologii." Moscow *Medicina*.

Korotaeva, N., A. Piruzyan, and I. Kosunskaya. 1/2014. *Individualnyj podchod k terapii akne: sistemnye preparaty.* Gaggenau, Germany: Kosmetik International.

Lighter, P. 2012. "Vosstanovitselnaya posloynaya terapiya." *Kosmeticheskiy forum.* www.reface.co.il.

Lighter, P. 4/2015. *Biomechanika litsa: myslim systemno.* Les Nouvelles Esthetiques Ukraine.

Lighter, P. 3/2016. *Forma opredelyaetsya funktsiey.* Les Nouvelles Esthetiques Ukraine.

Meder, T., and Y. Zubcova. 2015. "Beauty Myths." *Alpina Digital.*

Melnik, B. C. 2011. *Evidence for Acne-promoting Effects of Milk and Other Insulinotropic Dairy Products.* Nestle Nutrition workshop Ser Pediatr Program.

Mihaylova, N. 3/2013. *Staraya Problema – Novoe reshenie.* Les Nouvelles Esthetiques.

Nestor, M. S. 2011. "Duration of Action of AbobotulinumtoxinA and Onabotulinum-toxinA." *Journal of Clinical and Aesthetic Dermatology* 4 (9): 43–49.

Norat, T., L. Dossus, S. Rinaldi, and Others. 2007. "Diet, Serum Insulin-like Growth Factor- I and IGF-binding Protein-3 in European Women." *European Journal of Clinical Nutrition* 61 (1): 91–98.

Obagi, Z. E. 2014a. *The Art of Skin Health Restoration and Rejuvenation.* 2nd edn. London: CRC Press.

Obagi, Z. E. 2014b. *Rosacea.* UK: Body Language, 2014. www.bodylanguage.net/rosacea/. Accessed May 12, 2014.

Potemkina, M. 1/2015. *Kombinirovannaya metodika esteticheskoy korrekcii kozhi oblasti zhivota*. Gaggenau, Germany: Kosmetik International.

Rich-Edwards, J. W., D. Ganmaa, M. N. Pollak, E. K. Nakamoto, K. Kleinman, U. Tserendolgor, W. C. Willett, and A. L. Frazier. 2007. "Milk Consumption and the Prepubertal Somatotropic Axis." *Nutrition Journal* 6:28.

Sanchez, N. P., M. A. Pathak, S. Sato, T. B. Fitzpatrick, J. L. Sanchez, and M. C. Mihm Jr. 1981. "Melasma: A Clinical, Light Microscopic, Ultrastructural, and Immunofluorescence Study." *Journal of the American Academy of Dermatology* 4 (6): 698–710.

Sokolova, E. 1/2015. *Zhirovye otlozheniya v oblasti sedmogo sheynogo pozvonka*. Gaggenau, Germany: Kosmetik International.

Starkova, E. 1/2014. *Mezoniti: nastoyaschee I buduschee*. Gaggenau, Germany: Kosmetik International.

Strauss, J. S., D. P. Krowchuk, J. J. Leyden, A. W. Lucky, A. R. Shalita, E. C. Siegfried, D. M. Thiboutot, A. S. Van Voorhees, K. A. Beutner, C. K. Sieck, R. Bhushan, and American Academy of Dermatology/ American Academy of Dermatology Association. 2007. "Guidelines of Care for Acne Vulgaris Management." *Journal of the American Academy of Dermatology* 56 (4): 651–63.

Tan, J. K., K. Vasey, and K. Y. Fung. 2001. "Benefits and Perceptions of Patients with Acne." *Journal of American Academy of Dermatology* 44 (3): 439–45.

Tomasello, D. M. 2016. *Winning Skin: The Anti-aging Path to Looking and Feeling Younger.* Milwaukee: The Medical College of Wisconsin.

Unna, P. 1896. *The Histopathology of Disease of the Skin.* New York: Macmillan and Co.

Varich, M. 2014. *Gyperpigmentatsiya periorbital-noy zony: pravila terapii.* Gaggenau, Germany: Kosmetik International.

Vashkevich, M. 1/2012. *Uspeshnoe sochetanie: RF-lifting + inekcionnye metody.* Gaggenau, Germany: Kosmetik International.

Vashkevich, M., I. Belenkaya, and K. Levit. 3/2012. *Pozitivnyj Reaction.* Greece: CosmoMed.

Volkova, S. 2014. *Tredlifting & Biorevitalizatsiya verchney treti litsa: opyt kombinirovannogo primeneniya.* Gaggenau, Germany: Kosmetik International.

Wilkin, J., M. Dahl, M. Detmar, L. Drake, A. Feinstein, R. Odom, and F. Powell. 2002. "Standard Classification of Rosacea: Report of the National Rosacea Society Expert Committee on the Classification and Staging of Rosacea. *Journal of the American Academy of Dermatology* 46 (4): 584–7.

Williams, H. C., R. P. Dellavalle, and S. Garner. 2012. "Acne Vulgaris." *Lancet* 379 (9813): 361–72.

Wiseman, A. 2013. *Skin Deep Soul 7 Inc.* Canada: Jannet Matthews.

Zimina, E. V. 4/2011. *Melanotsity.* Greece: Cosmomed.

Zorina, A. 1/2014. *Kletochnye technologii v kosmetologii: perspektivy primeneniya.* Gaggenau, Germany: Kosmetik International.

72714234R00110

Made in the USA
San Bernardino, CA
29 March 2018